Watch out for burnout

Watch out for burnout

a look at its signs, prevention, and cure

DONALD E.
DEMARAY

BAKER BOOK HOUSE
Grand Rapids, Michigan 49506

ISBN: 0-8010-2930-9

Printed in the United States of America

First printing, July 1983
Second printing, December 1983
Third printing, April 1984

to
Kathleen
faithful at every point

Contents

Acknowledgments

Gratitude, in the first instance, goes to those persons in North America, South Africa, and Great Britain, who graciously shared knowledge and experience, and opened my eyes to some of the crucial concerns and therapies relative to burnout. Everywhere I found people eager and willing to talk. Ministers in all three countries completed my survey research instrument on fitness. Without the contributions of many, I would not have undertaken this project.

The concern I sensed in interviewing dozens of people over several years gave birth to research and writing. My prayer is that many will learn to spot signs of burnout and discover how to avoid it, and that those suffering through the experience will see lights to lead them to personal and professional renewal.

I must record thanks to the Officers of Administration, Asbury Theological Seminary, Frank Bateman Stanger, past President of the Seminary and former chairman of the Officers. I must also express thanks to the Seminary's committee responsible for recommending sabbaticals to the Officers, Kenneth Kinghorn, chairman; Louis Caister, secretary.

To Principal Philip Capp of the Evangelical Bible Seminary of Southern Africa, to his wife Carmena and their delightfully inquisitive daughter Karen, go further thanks for stimulation, information, and permission to use books in their family library. I must include thanks for access to the Seminary library. The Seminary faculty and staff proved themselves solidly supportive, most particularly Professor and Mrs. James Kopp, Professor Beth Beckelhymer, and the Seminary secretary known simply and affectionately as Olive.

The following libraries, in addition to those listed above, opened their doors to me: the new Barbican Library specializing in the arts, Barbican Center, London; the British Museum Reading Room; the British Museum Drawings and Antiquities Room; the Oak Hill Theological College library, London; the London Borough of Enfield Public Libraries, Southgate Circus and DeBohun branches; the Public Library, Pietermaritzburg, South Africa. I want also to thank Principal David Wheaton of London's Oak Hill Theological College for access to his private library; and William David Faupel, Acting Director of Library Services, Asbury Theological Seminary, for courtesies.

I wish to express appreciation to key persons who gave time and encouragement to me in the course of the research and writing. David McKenna, present President of Asbury Theological Seminary; Pastor John Waterman of the Evangelical Church of High Barnet, London, and his warmhearted congregation; Dr. James Moss, professor in the University of London; my parents, C. Dorr and Grace Demaray; David and Margaret Field of Oak Hill College; Tony and Sharon Casurella, Birkenhead, England; and to my dear wife who read the entire manuscript and made suggestions only a wife can make.

Prologue

Persons of all vocations suffer burnout. A recent study of one seminary's alumni indicated that burnout most often happened five years after graduation. Another research shows American schoolteachers burn out between the fifth and the sixth years of service. An earlier study of teachers (1978) points to burnout after ten years.

Multiple causes account for dropout, but studies show acute fatigue one significant dynamic. The current duration-of-service norm for inner-city social workers and inner-city lawyers turns out to be only two years. One stateside psychiatrist says 50 percent of his clients are missionaries. A long-time missionary comments that a typical overseas worker lasts five to six years. A large denomination reports losses of a thousand clergy annually.

Homemakers go through burnout too. Marriages often run into difficulty after five years. Boredom and depression are not uncommon in families.

We need to do something to cope with burnout. The first priority is to recognize the signals. Signs of oncoming burn-out, documented by experienced counselors, include a dim-inution of enthusiasm, gray feelings, negativity, withdrawal, lowering of competence, absenteeism, sluggish thinking, and anger. As burnout deepens, disgust, paralysis, radical iso-lation, full-scale depression, and inability to plan and work may appear.

How do we deal with this multi-factorial phenomenon called burnout? First, enlist the help of significant persons (authority figures) who listen and offer genuine acceptance. Any sign however subtle of rejection only advances the sense of helplessness. The victim already knows shame and guilt feelings.

Attacking burnout sometimes means a job change; so that the necessary fresh perspective may emerge. Prayer at depth level, along with a workable recovery program (not always drugs), becomes a welcome therapy.

Unhurried time with family, full-scale recreation, and ad-equate sleep are imperatives. Modern research demonstrates that physical and emotional problems may stem from poor nutrition. Adjusting lifestyle to a slower pace, confiding in a trusted friend, systematic physical exercise, absorbing hob-bies, may function as effective instruments of healing.

Humor proves itself a powerful remedy and preventative. John Milton intuited something of this:

> Sport that wrinkled care derides,
> And laughter holding both his sides,
> Come, and trip it as ye go
> On the light fantastic toe.

Whatever the prescription, the aim is to find Edwin Mark-ham's "place of central calm" at the "heart of the cyclone tearing the sky." To help people find a core of peace is the target of this book.

In this book help comes packaged in digestable units. Sin-gle meditations relate causes and find cures. Thirteen crucial areas of cause and cure provide the framework of informa-tion and exploration. Your invitation is to enter into seven contemplation experiences for each of the thirteen concern areas. The meditational approach stimulates search, prayer, intentionality, and fruitful dialog with family and friends. Best of all, it opens one to the dynamically fresh work of the Holy Spirit.

Donald E. Demaray
London, England

1

Burnout

A Burn-Out is "someone in a state of fatigue or frustration brought about by devotion to a cause, way of life, or relationship that failed to produce the expected reward."

Herbert J. Freudenberger
Burn-Out: The High Cost of High Achievement

What Is Burnout?

Herbert J. Freudenberger, psychoanalyst, invented the term *burnout* to describe his own experiences. Working in the Haight-Ashbury district of San Francisco in the 1960s, he grew severely disappointed. He operated a clinic for years, but could see little result. He saw countless persons daily in spite of his physical exhaustion and emotional drain. He never got to bed before one or two A.M.

In this condition one tends to negative thinking and depression. That negativity can take any number of expressions like irritability, cynicism, gossip, anger, rigidity, pessimism, or unwillingness to listen. Burnout results from overintensity in

13

goal achievement. Every moment must be invested. Push, push, push is the way of life. Only unbendingly high expectations, really a kind of perfectionism, can answer this awful drive.

The disjunction between ideal and real is inadmissable to the burnout victim. This attitude becomes difficult for a minister who holds high moral ideals for his young people, but sees them caught in the clutches of sin. Or for a doctor who cannot alleviate the suffering of his patients. Or for a social worker who finally gets money to help someone only to have it refused.

Youthful idealism yields to life's brutalities. How does one live with that? One can clam up and withdraw, protecting himself momentarily from hurt. One can cut him/herself off from full participation, thus depriving oneself of liberated joy. One can make of him/herself a battering ram, persisting while getting hurt more and damaging others.

But there are better ways. Dr. Freudenberger fought burnout creatively. He wrote on burnout describing causes and cures. He spent more time with his family. He even stayed home during vacations instead of trying to use every spare hour to cure the ills of mankind. He moved to New York for a fresh lease on life and his profession. He would not entertain defeat. He found a way out.

How to Identify Burnout

Hallmarks of the burnout experience include boredom, frustration, domestic problems, hopelessness, a sense of helplessness about one's environment, rejection and paranoia, pessimism, stress, meaninglessness, enervation, irritability. All of us have some of these feelings some of the time, especially after heavy duty like a major deadline, moving from one community to another, arranging a public event. A good day or two off usually takes care of the exhaustion and we're ready for life again.

Chronic weariness can sneak up. Before we know it we can tire readily. We find chatter annoying, go in circles with little to show for effort invested, turn sour on life, fight inner heaviness, snap at family and friends, isolate ourselves from routine social contacts, feel terribly harried, let important dates and facts skip from memory. We may even show psychosomatic distress—pain in the stomach, headaches, persistent sore throats.

When we cannot laugh, especially at ourselves, that's a pretty good sign something has gone wrong.

Teachers who invest in their students, only to be rejected, may suffer burnout. Young professionals who graduate under the illusion they can "handle everything," need warning flags waved in full view. The real world doesn't yield to quick and "competent" answers. When standards elude and goals evade us, we feel out of touch with things as they are. Life can deal its blows when we see little success.

If we can identify the marks and causes of burnout, we can also find some cures. The people who really take a day or two off after a big event have part of the secret. So do those who eat good food, sleep well, talk with God, dialog with spouse and friends. Those who slow down and define success realistically have found a cure.

Why Me?

Because of your total commitment.

We are taught in church and school to give ourselves totally to God and our work, but even that truth needs to be put in perspective. Jesus never lost sleep because He couldn't preach outside the Palestinian strip. He called Paul and his friends to do that. Jesus did not win all His disciples. His own brothers refused to believe in Him until after the resurrection. Jesus did not fret Himself about all this; He left family and friends in the hands of His sovereign Father.

Jesus ministered within the framework of His own style. He never allowed anyone to dictate how He went about His mission. He was true to Himself. He did not allow persons or society to define commitment for Him. He and His Father made the definitions.

How do you define total commitment? Society often describes it as overachieving. Our culture creates compulsive persons with a perfectionistic streak, people who have to change the world.

Have we forgotten that only God knows how to change the world? Recognize Him as omniscient, all-knowing. Let Him determine your own personal role in changing the world. Refuse to allow your societally conditioned and outsized drive to determine your role. When He assigns, work in His strength. Sincere plodders often achieve more in a lifetime than fiery men and women who burn out prematurely.

Had Elijah lived in contemporary America, he might have been a coronary Type A. Type A behavior is defined as "an action-emotion complex that can be observed in any person who is aggressively involved in a chronic incessant struggle to achieve more and more in less and less time, and if required to do so, against the opposing efforts of other things or other persons." One study revealed that 50 percent of American males fall into this type of behavior. Dollars, things, numbers of people and buildings, goals, deadlines—anything at all that shows "success" documents total commitment.

We are not surprised to learn that this produces chronic stress which triggers high blood pressure, unwanted cholesterol, heart attack, even diabetes. Because Type A behavior is learned, it can also be unlearned. That's the good news.

Evidently Elijah had to unlearn stressful living. He learned it the hard way. The Bible pictures him as a speed runner, hard-hitting prophet, inspired faith builder, rugged outdoors-man, triumphant challenger. Overintense, overachieving, he paid the price as we shall see. We shall also notice how he found renewal, fresh meaning in life, and a recovered sense of God's presence.

Elijah's "Peak" Experience

D. G. Kehl, in an article for *Christianity Today* (Nov. 20, 1981), "Burnout: The Risk of Reaching Too High," rightly observes that burnout may come after "peak" experiences. Like Elijah's Mt. Carmel victory.

Imagine the prophet's emotional investment with half a thousand pagan prophets pitted against him; the enormous test of his faith; the dynamic flow of events; the tense dialog; the climax of fire falling and consuming the sacrifice, wood, stone and water! This whole experience would naturally take its emotional and spiritual toll, even from one who had strong religious orientation.

Great crises drain human beings. Elijah's let-down ranged from the "all gone" feeling, to lethargy and melancholia (I Kings 19).

Some authors say their great let-downs follow the completion of writing projects. Internal conflicts rage while the mind rushes into dark and discolored alleyways. Why didn't I write a better book? Surely this publication will give rise to rejection. The research will prove inadequate.

Writers like all creators must wait for their emotions to return to normal. They reject the raging inner conflict by letting time do its magic. They must rest from the intense enthusiasm required to bring a fresh creation to completion.

Mission accomplished means glands no longer provide energy to match the challenge, the search for stimuli to gen-

17

erate productivity comes to a standstill. One's world view alters as reentry takes place.

Wise achievers (1) expect let-down and plan for it, (2) keep their cool during and immediately after reentry, and (3) refurbish body, mind, and spirit by relaxation, diversion, and worship.

Handling Rejection

Jezebel informed Elijah she would wipe him out within twenty-four hours. Most of us will not experience rejection in such radical form, but the prophet did and the result was a chain of negative thoughts that made him feel worthless.

Rejection sets up an inner dialog that spells self-doubt. We fear that people have only tolerated us, that in reality we just haven't "made it." This persistent negative thinking leads to depression.

No wonder Elijah withdrew to the wilderness. The act was both wise and symptomatic. We admire the man who prior to isolation had played the game with all his might. Some never get on life's stage because they don't want to risk themselves.

Nathaniel Hawthorne dreamed of writing a play but it never materialized. The outline, discovered in the papers he left, shows clearly the possibilities of the plot. The play's development might have proved fascinating because the chief character never once appears.

Elijah did not do his thing in a corner, hidden and protected from the possibilities of rejection. He got out there on the stage and played his part though his critics shot him down.

How do we handle rejection before it draws us into the abyss of depression? (1) Deal with the real anger. Rejection's hurt is the obverse side of anger. (2) Having faced rejection deal with your unreleased emotions by playing a fast game of racketball, jogging, chopping or hauling wood, throwing yourself into just about any wholesome activity. You aim to use up the adrenalin. (3) Develop defenses like humor. Virtually every rejection has its funny side and wit has a way of dissolving the impact. (4) Always pray for grace to love your rejector, who really projects his own frustrations through his behavior.

Elijah Recovers from Depression

Elijah's rejection and resulting anger developed into depression. Fear gripped him, isolation came next, suicidal thoughts tormented him, terrible all-aloneness bore in on him.

I Kings 19 carries not only the story of Elijah's black emotions, but also the parallel account of God's therapy. Elijah calls on God, agonizing, "It is enough; now, Lord, take away my life; for I am no better than my fathers." Then the defeated man escaped in sleep to awake at the touch of an angel: "Arise and eat." After eating and drinking, he fell asleep again. The angel woke him a second time to eat and drink.

During the next forty days Elijah traveled to Horeb where he took lodging in a cave, a fitting spot for his darkened spirit. God spoke: "What are you doing here, Elijah?" Elijah's answer betrays his bitterness, egotism, and paranoia: People don't appreciate me.

The Lord tried more radical therapy. Summoning Elijah to His presence on Mount Horeb, God sent a great and terrible wind that split rocks open. ". . . but the Lord was not in the wind."

Then God caused a powerful earthquake, ". . . but the

Lord was not in the earthquake." Next came a searing fire, ". . . but the Lord was not in the fire." None of these shock treatments worked. God remained a closed book to the depressed man.

God's fourth communication, "a still small voice," penetrated Elijah's self-absorbed mind. At first the message proved too painful, and the prophet returned to his cave. "What are you doing here, Elijah?" Bitterness, egocentricity, and paranoia answered. Nobody's good but me, and people want to kill me.

Now the Lord brought therapy to its climax: "Go and do. . . ." Elijah's assignment: the anointing of two kings and the ordination of a young prophet.

Therapy came in God's presence, loving patience, and purposeful assignments. Elijah's sense of personal worth was restored.

Face Fatigue

Elijah does not appear to have faced his fatigue. He tried several ways to avoid reality. Consider two of them.

They lie at opposite ends of a continuum. Escape is at one end and overactivity at the other. One says, "Resign everything." Elijah dropped work and human beings, even his personal servant. The other extreme announces, "Drown weariness in busyness." To get away is good; to exercise is good; but is mile after mile of exhausting hikes in wilderness and desert really desirable? Both ends of the continuum signal danger.

A young husband walking away from his lovely wife and children comments: "I feel trapped." Close examination reveals an overcrowded schedule. He had achieved success professionally and personally. Fatigue set in long before the surprise exit. He overextended himself until something had to let go—in this case, wife and family.

The dialog between Elijah and God was therapy which eventuated in clarity of thought and rational action. The young husband and father should have talked with God and his family. Unvented interpersonal tensions are dynamite. Talk provides catharsis; dialog opens windows on fresh perspective. This can furnish hope and new possibilities.

Standing up to one's fatigue is neither antisocial isolation nor inordinate involvement, but the designation of authentic priorities. This happy equilibrium comes with liberated exploration filled with love and imagination, the same context in which God works.

2
God's Healing

I believe He [Jesus] was demonstrating that if we can find what wholeness or salvation is all about, healing and physical well-being will be a by-product.

Bruce Larson
There's a Lot More to Health Than Not Being Sick

Our Center and Source of Healing

Carl Jung got to the heart of healing when he shared his research conclusion that health comes by contact with a meaningful center of reality. Jung believed that truly religious patients get well faster while sick people without religious orientation tend to stay sick.

Push God out of the center, and confusion infiltrates our minds. Hearts that are made for God exist in restless anxiety without Him. The inner vacuum tailored for God Himself balks at substitutes. This explains why surrender to God, recognition of Him as crowned King of our universe, brings instant peace. This peace of adjustment is the reverse of maladjustment which is burnout.

23

Peace *(shalom)* really means wholeness, well-being. The biblical word is *salvation.* The Scriptures teach that *shalom* comes from God who resides in righteous hearts. When one lives in harmony with the Creator and His goals, peace follows. Jesus, the Prince of Peace (health), came to demonstrate that law.

How do we get into sync with God? (1) Cooperate with what Jung saw as an instinctive drive of the psyche toward health. Cooperation lies in identification with God. (2) Recognize the true source of integration. Bifurcation, indeed proliferation, results from God-substitute attempts. (3) Avoid all hints of religious faith not authenticated by God Himself. Many knowing Jung's law of health try foreign deities. Sooner or later the liberating truth gets through: *only God fits.* (4) Open yourself to growth. Some discover reality only to stay for life with that earliest discovery. God is very big. Abundant living flows toward great goals, introducing new experience and fresh insight. These rewards generate wholeness.

Carl Jung points to the core of healing—God Himself.

Healing in the Rat Race?

"Whereas there were 10 components per silicon chip in 1960, increasing to several hundred by 1970, by 1976 there were 10,000 and a year later over 30,000. Very large-scale integration (VLSI) will bring the production of microcircuits to an equivalent of 100,000 on a chip, which is less than the size of your fingernail, by 1981, and one million components on a quarter-inch square chip are forecast for the mid 1980s. The advent of the microprocessor . . . now means that a wide range of . . . skills can be extended or even displaced." (Morris Maddocks, *The Christian Healing Ministry.*)

We gulp breathlessly at fast-paced developments. Our

world expands and compresses at the same time. Concordes take three hours to cross the Atlantic; dishlike disks open our TV screens to France as easily as the hometown channels. We travel fast physically, visually, and viscerally. The whirl of activity gives us guilt feelings as does escape from it all. No wonder Bishop Michael Ramsey observes, ". . . souls are starved by activism."

Sometimes we cry, "O Lord, why Silicon Valley? Why the micro- and macro-electronics revolution? Is there no release from this burned-out feeling that comes from the constant bombardment of stimuli?"

Some get by with mild psychosomatic reactions like tinnitus, ringing in the ears. Others respond more radically, the tinnitus developing into almost unbearable inner pounding.

A young English pastor calls his alma mater from his hospital bed. Would a staff member please come to see him? Gladly an administrator comes but the pastor's comments do not reflect much happiness.

"I cannot stand the noise in this hospital," the patient complains. "My blood pressure stays high. Kidney failure can come any moment. So can cardiac arrest." Deep concerns tumble out, "Drugs help, but their side effects frighten me."

The college staff member lays hands on the young pastor and prays. Almost immediately well-being replaces anxieties. Healing, now initiated, takes hold and progresses day by day. Perspective returns when parish problems are reduced to size. God takes control once more. Burnout translates into God's gracious gift of wholeness.

The Renewing Power of the Holy Spirit

When we allow God-substitutes into our lives (how subtly that happens), we have the powerful therapeutic resource of confession. With real confession comes assurance of sins for-

25

given and the consequent renewal of the Holy Spirit. St. Jerome, writing in the fourth century from his own ecclesiastical setting, told of the renewal of confession. Pastors lay their hands on the sinners and ask for the return of the Holy Spirit.

Healing can take place only when imbedded sin comes to the surface to be cleansed away. Healing prayers can facilitate getting at those sins. The penitent sufferer finds immense release. Reconciliation is powerful therapy, getting at the root of things as medications may not. (Prescription drugs may only cover disease causes.) Courageously face the causes of your burnout feelings.

We can know daily renewing of the Spirit by sincere prayers. Praying the Lord's Prayer has great potential for spiritual rejuvenation. St. Augustine saw the daily saying of the Lord's Prayer as "a daily baptism."

The preacher of the Gospel offers his people the hope of forgiveness only after he himself experiences fresh cleansing. Newly filled with the Spirit, the anointed minister enters the pulpit to declare the mighty therapeutic acts of God. His own therapy is thereby deepened, strengthened, advanced and sealed. Preaching may serve as profound catharsis for a preacher struggling against burnout.

Tragic is the preacher who does not face his own and his people's sins. Glorious with resurrection power is the church which owns its simulated gods, hands them over to the real deity of the universe, and leaves with the joy of the Lord which is strength.

Someone has accurately observed that "there is no reconstruction or healing of the human personality more complete than that which Christ's forgiveness provides."

Answers to Pain

Pain has four aspects: physical, mental, social and spiritual. Some types of malignancy inflict little or no physical pain, but the mental agony can be great. In terminal disease, the sense of isolation may prove to be the real pain. People shun the presence of death and avoid the apprehensions created by social norms. For one who lives with unresolved tensions, pain multiplies. Burnout is a species of unresolved tension. Pain and physical discomfort often accompany it.

What answers can we give?

The immediate family must rally to furnish a support system strong as an army with banners. The strengthening nourishment of close loved ones literally relieves pain. Because none of the four types of pain can divorce itself from any others, when one undergoes treatment for a specific pain, other coexistent pain may also be modified. Family affirmation can relieve burnout pain and accompanying physical pain.

Talk freely and openly to a godly person. Sensitive listeners permit people to say whatever they wish. They also allow material to come out at its own rate. They never force insight, knowing that comes from the Holy Spirit, the ultimate therapist. A burnout in pain will talk to an easy listener; besides, natural sharing builds an atmosphere that says "therapy materializes in relationship."

Ask for the laying-on-of-hands with oil, as the Scriptures instruct. Invite the elders of your local church (people you can trust) to join in the service of Christian healing. Prepare yourself by asking God to clear away obstructions to the flow of His divine medicine. You may take Holy Communion as part of the preparation. Pain often goes after a service of Christian healing.

Ask your prayer group to sustain you in intercession. An established, intimate group of believers who talk comfortably about spiritual concerns is the free-flowing vehicle of enormous spiritual power. Take advantage of this potential for the release of the Spirit.

The rules for the management of pain apply to the full range of suffering: depression, oppression, inhibitions, physical fatigue, emotional exhaustion, domestic problems, interpersonal conflicts. Christian resources hold many answers to pain.

Counseling to Heal

Whether one counsels the burnout or seeks counsel to free himself, true healing principles find their roots in God. What shape does theologically rooted counseling take?

Availability. God does not keep a date book. Good counselors project interested availability. Persons in need can open themselves to the active grace of Christ. Never in a hurry, counselor and counselee allow God's Spirit to work as He will.

Listen. God hears. We listen with our ears to hear the raw outline of the problem; we listen with intuition to fill in what is unspoken; we listen with the heart to bring experience and memory to bear on the situation; we listen with the spirit to attune ourselves to God's answer.

Vulnerability. God opened Himself to the cross through Christ. Therapy comes only when we risk. To protect ourselves from sin only erects barriers and creates false securities bound to collapse. God helps those who level with Him. God works through counselors who admit their inadequacies.

Surrender. God's basic spiritual law is surrender. To pretend we can solve problems is sheer folly and unpragmatic. The character of today's complex concerns overwhelms our unaided abilities. Moreover, when we focus on our problems too long we only accentuate them; when we tell God we haven't answers He provides healing. "The Church," says Bishop Morris Maddocks, "is not in business as a problem solver. Its job is to see that problems are surrendered to him who alone can make all things new."

Intercession. Jesus intercedes for us. Prayer in the counseling setting, marked by the Presence, gives assurance from the only real source of assurance. The call to obedience comes through with sharp specificity in authentic prayer. Praise, joy, anticipation, and total trust characterize effective intercession. Counselor and counselee sense God alive in the power of the resurrected Lord.

Caring for the Newly Healed

Convalescence, like physical recovery, is also needed in spiritual recuperation. Integration into the Body of Christ is the first step to wholeness and stabilization. Worship and work, powerful twin therapies, open doors to prayer, love, and meaning.

One of the big challenges facing today's Church is frontiering fresh ways to get convalescents into the life of the local believing group. Scripture, praise, and preaching are pharmaceutically active. We require a new perspective on the implemented Gospel that will unleash the medicinal potential available in Christ.

Surely the prayer group movement supersedes stale, ritualistic prayer meetings. The fresh breezes of body life worship unfreeze dormant longings. We have yet to come to the New Testament *koinonia,* uncalculating and spontaneously inclusive in its contacts and outreach. What will facilitate the development of this early Church fellowship?

The recovery of therapeutic preaching. Even modern secular psychiatrists call for preaching that faces sin, shows the cure in forgiveness, and assures hearers of security-in-depth.

The recovery of worship in the Spirit. A worship with substance. A worship that sends people home on wings, not flat tires. The dynamic? Scripture saturation and prayer preparation.

The recovery of community. Dr. and Mrs. Michael Daves opened their home and dinner table to Kathleen and me after an all-night flight. The warmth, openness, laughter, and joy that permeated the atmosphere of their English home, rested us. "Do return. We covet the chance to get better acquainted." Nothing was put on; there was genuine, excited sincerity. We left saying, "That is a Christian home, a model." God's Spirit gives birth to the flow of soul which is community.

Preaching, worship, and community have great power not only to prevent and cure burnout, but also to give stability to those newly recovered.

Resurrection

The final healing comes with death. That healing begins before the cessation of earthly life. Modern thanatological research, built in part on explorations of clinical death experiences, shows the liberations that eventuate as heaven comes nearer.

Freedom from self in the body. The dying one, divorced from the body, can observe the doctors, nurses, technicians, and activities. We are told it is not a frightening experience to look down on the whole drama.

The fast-moving cinema. One's life passes in view with pictures flowing selectively to the truly significant experiences. Contributions are reevaluated as one learns which involvements truly counted. Only God knows the genuinely important.

New vision. Going through the tunnel to the next world of brilliant light, vivid color, intense reality, and exquisite joy sometimes includes the sight of loved ones and friends. This proves so unspeakably fulfilling that the departing wish to move right into heaven. Those who return to their bodies often bring a resurrection wholeness that is deeply life-changing.

God returns these experienced people to give us a glimpse of the glorious existence ahead. That shared knowledge carries its own healing transforming power.

The vision is part of the spiritual world a Christian experiences in some measure. The awareness enlarges with time. Conversion, fresh fillings of the Spirit, repeated celebrations of the Lord's Supper, insightful preaching, the emerging awareness of hymn meanings represent accumulated revelation which partakes of heaven.

We can even articulate a formula that the deeper and wider our awareness is of God and His world, the nearer to resurrection wholeness we come. Clear perception of this experiential fact gives us strong stability in fatigue and provides the sure knowledge of coming renewal.

3

The Healing Power of Humor

. . . the sense of humour I have found of use in every single occasion of my life.

Katherine Mansfield

Humor's Source

Joy is the origin of the Christian's spirit of humor. "In the world you have tribulation," Jesus said with characteristic candor, "but, be of good cheer, I have overcome the world." The psalmist talks of God's anointing "with the oil of gladness" (45:7; cf. Heb. 1:9).

In this joy lies real strength: ". . . the joy of the LORD is your strength" (Neh. 8:10b). Psalm 16:11 tells us that in God's presence "there is fulness of joy" and "pleasures for evermore."

Agnes Sanford discovered the relationship between joy and prayer in connection with the healing of her baby. Ill six weeks, the little one did not mend despite Mrs. Sanford's earnest intercessions. Then a young pastor came to pray. She thought his prayers would do no good, but he insisted.

When he prayed holding the baby in his arms, "light shone in his eyes. I believed. For joy is the heavenly 'okay' of the inner life of power. . . ." The baby fell asleep and awakened healed.

Reflecting on her earlier prayers, Agnes Sanford wisely observed that she had allowed fear and desperation to grip her heart. These negatives had blocked her intercessions.

When Katherine Mansfield said "the sense of humour I have found of use in every single occasion of my life," she pointed to a basic law of successful living. We can pray over a crucial issue or seek a way to relate meaningfully to others and ourselves. God's gift of joy, from which laughter springs, oils the hinges so we can open windows onto new light and see answers rich with possibilities.

When the flag waves over Buckingham Palace, Elizabeth II's London home, the Queen is in residence. When joy writes itself on a person's face, the Holy Spirit is in residence. When laughter spills over and tumbles like a waterfall, we know the joyous Spirit within is working therapeutically against the threat of burnout.

Laughter Is Therapeutic

Laughter is medicine. Norman Cousins discovered this for himself. Home from a working trip in Russia, he ended up in the hospital exhausted and very ill. Tests revealed he had a rare terminal disease. Fortunately the doctor was flexible, and the two men, Dr. Hitzig and Mr. Cousins, tailored a therapy program.

Cousins moved out of the hospital for privacy. He put into gear the full exercise of affirmative emotions to enhance his body chemistry. The crucial decision was to laugh a lot. Not that laughing proved easy: "Nothing is less funny than being flat on your back, with all the bones in your spine and joints hurting."

He met the pain challenge by systematically induced laughter. He began with Allen Funt's "Candid Camera" films, and went on to the Marx Brothers' flicks. "It worked. I made the joyous discovery that ten minutes of genuine belly laughter had an anesthetic effect and would give me at least two hours of pain-free sleep."

Cousins goes on: "When the pain-killing effect of the laughter wore off, we would switch on the motion-picture projector again, and, not infrequently, it would lead to another pain-free sleep interval." Sometimes the nurse read from humor books such as E. G. and Katherine White's *Subtreasury of American Humor* and Max Eastman's *The Enjoyment of Laugher.*

Did laughing really change his body chemistry? Was he actually getting well? Cousins answers ". . . we took sedimentation rate readings just before as well as several hours after the laughter episodes. Each time, there was a drop of at least five points. The drop by itself was not substantial, but it held and was cumulative."

Cousins' final conclusion? "I was greatly elated by the discovery that there is a physiologic basis for the ancient theory that laughter is good medicine."

The whole story can be found in the fascinating book by Norman Cousins, *Anatomy of an Illness.* There he gives the full range of rich details connected with his successful therapy. Laughter played its role in Cousins' cure. Surely it can help heal burnout and act as a preventative on a daily basis.

The Relaxation Response

The surrendered person lives at liberty to take life in stride and to laugh at himself.

Dr. James Moss, professor of orthodontics and head of his

department at the University of London's college of dentistry, packs an immense amount of work into his life. He is past president of the National Society of Orthodontists, and currently president of the European division of a world orthodontics association. He travels the globe presiding at meetings and sharing knowledge from his own surgical and research experiences.

Often people ask, "James, how do you do it all?" His reply comes as easily as his work: "I just do it. I don't take myself seriously. People wear masks," he comments. "They try to be perfect; they work so hard to get to the top. I don't care whether I get to the top."

There we have his secret, "I don't care whether I get to the top." He says, "I'm just myself."

He is. Everybody feels comfortable around him. He wastes no energy wearing a mask. Thus liberated, he serves with abandon not only as a dental surgeon and professor, but also as father and husband, and as elder and lay preacher.

How do we stop taking ourselves with undue seriousness? How do we get rid of the I've-got-to-make-it-to-the-top hangup which contributes to burnout?

The cartoonist's calling is to help us laugh at ourselves, to take away the onus of awful "must-ness." Pogo and Peanuts have great therapeutic potential. So do humorists like P.G. Wodehouse. No doubt one reason he lived so long is that he relaxed so much with laughter and pleasantry. The London *Times* hailed him a comic genius, recognized in his lifetime as a classic and an old master of farce. He died at ninety-three, Valentine's Day, 1975.

A good laugh may clear away early burnout feelings as morning sun burns off fog at the airport so the jets can take off.

Martin L. Gross, past editor of *Book Digest*, asked Erma Bombeck, "What does humor do for a person?"

Aunt Erma's reply is near classic: "It does everything. It could save your life. It really could, particularly when you're faced with a situation that you think you just cannot handle.

We've had that in our marriage situations 'Oh, . . . we're never going to survive this.' And then the humor comes back and says, 'Hey, we're going to be OK.' "

The Best Way to Be Serious

"The best way to get serious," says an insightful man, "is to get humorous." He illustrates his point in the context of public speech. "If you want an audience to take your message to heart, get them first to laugh." Laughter has a way of getting under our skin.

Laughter does more. It serves as a remarkably effective instrument for achieving dead serious goals. Humor puts people at ease in an atmosphere that gives birth to easy competence. Laughter triggers the flow of creative juices and puts the pieces of a puzzle together.

Without humor, driving seriousness becomes malignant. A wise elder missionary statesman said to a fledgling missionary, "If you want to live awhile out here in Africa, learn to see the funny side of life." *Reader's Digest* has a point when it bills laughter as the "best medicine."

I asked a university president the secret of his longevity. "Humor," came the one-word reply. Humor enables him to carry his burdens lightly.

Humor allows us to live with the contradictions of life. The man who must always act rationally kills himself with intensity. He will embarrass himself by his own contradictory behavior. People laugh at his over-seriousness, but he cannot laugh at himself. To laugh at one's inconsistency reveals the deepest consistency. That's why Art Buchwald makes us double up with hilarity.

Humor allows us to live comfortably with ourselves—one significant clue to avoiding burnout. Perfectionism is the worst kind of seriousness, a poison that brings death to liberty and rigor mortis to the spirit. Humor is the antibiotic that heals the terribly perfect, thus releasing the inner man, restoring perspective, and turning creativity on once more.

Sir James Barrie (Peter Pan, Act I) tells us the origin of fairies: "When the first baby laughed for the first time, the laugh broke into a thousand pieces and they all went skipping about, and that was the beginning of fairies." In the same Act, Sir James comments, "Every time a child says, 'I don't believe in fairies' there is a little fairy somewhere that falls down dead." Laughter gives rebirth to the fairy child in us all.

Psychologists remind us how important it is to keep that child alive. The child within is freshness, wonder, excitement, and the faith that accomplishes the impossible. Super-seriousness robs us of that child. "Do you believe in fairies?" asks Sir James Barrie in Act IV: "If you believe, clap your hands!"

How can serious adults facing the threat of burnout believe once more? Listen to Jesus about becoming a little child to enter the Kingdom of wholeness. See Him throw off the weight of Pharasaic criticism by the figure of speech "you white-washed walls." Surely the common people broke up in sidesplitting laughter and heard Him gladly. Hear Him talk about "the beam in the eye" as he uncovers the gross imperfections of people posing as perfect. Elton Trueblood found so much humor in Jesus that he wrote a whole book about it.

Jesus was as serious as any man who ever lived. It's possible to achieve serious goals without the over-intensity that contributes to burnout.

Humor Greases the Wheels

"Not many humor books here, I'm afraid," lamented the village librarian. She disappeared, returning in a few minutes with four or five books. She saw me forty minutes later visibly tickled as I read Morley and Leacock.

"Looks like you found something funny," she volunteered.

"Yes, and I'm trying to figure a way to check out these delightful books. I don't have my cards with me." Patiently she explained I would have to have the check-out cards. I smiled knowingly and went on reading.

"Of course," she added as an afterthought, "if you're desperate I can give you a Spring Bank Holiday emergency card."

"That would be nice," I replied to the gracious English lady, thinking, "Humor's atmosphere persuades as little else can."

The amusing Robert Morley volume is his *Book of Worries*, an alphabetically arranged listing of things that make us fret: age, baldness, blood pressure, cholesterol, clothes . . . dozens more. Any of these farcically funny short pieces can loosen our tensions and release our jets. The escaping steam will express itself in torrents of laughter. Guaranteed!

The Stephen Leacock piece, "My Financial Career," I had not seen since youth when I read it in *Reader's Digest*. Now I laughed harder, the years interpreting the story's subtle nuances. I read it to Kathleen at home and we both laughed till we cried. This little gem of an essay takes less than ten minutes to read, but furnishes a day's therapy.

Work comes easier after side-splitting humor. Machinery moves more smoothly. Hope makes its reentry quickly, quietly, almost unawares. Possibilities grow luminous. Artifice and therefore stress disappear.

When wheels squeak, apply the grease of humor.

A Way of Seeing

Humorists win. They win because they see with laughter-corrected vision.

A novelist probably determined the success of his career

because he used laughter as an agent for keeping his sight at 20/20. As a beginner reporter he got a letter from his father who wrote that his son would never amount to a hill of beans. Annoyed at his father, he wrote that ". . . at 21 he did indeed seem incapable, but he had in fact thought out his life goal. His plan for achievement? At 30 he intended to be a great newspaper reporter; at 40 a great editor; at 50 a great story writer; at 60 a great fiction writer; at 70 a great grandfather; at 80 a great admirer of beautiful women; at 90 a great loss to the community."

His father had a good laugh. Significantly the years saw the son's career proceed along the very lines he predicted in that delightful letter.

I have a friend who refuses to worry. He knows worry fogs his lenses and confuses focus. My friend fought big problems for forty years, but insisted on dissipating his worry potential in humor. Riotously funny, he reduces problems to a size easily seen then places them in a corner. He never allows them to tower over him so they can look down from some vague but apprehensive position. Humor becomes the spectacles through which he sees life. This way of seeing held him to faith and kept him collected through a long illness then successful surgery of his wife. She now enjoys perfect health and together they relish retirement in Christian service overseas and at home.

Says Irving Oyle, a medical doctor, "Positive, beautiful thoughts trigger the release of beneficial hormones in the body and these in turn help the body to heal itself." But, he says, "If you presume that you live in a hostile universe, the reaction to that presumption is what wears out your body. Faith," Dr. Oyle concludes, "creates the hormones that make you live longer."

And what generates faith? Prayer, affirmative thinking, positive achievement, and, of course, humor. How do you look at your world? If through hostile, paranoid eyes, you can change your lenses, God being your ophthalmologist.

A Weapon

The Bible says, "Anxiety in a man's heart weighs him down" (Prov. 12:25). Anxiety turns into specific fear of things that may happen to us. In turn when those very things do happen the Bible rightly claims that the things we fear come upon us (Job 3:25).

Humor is God's weapon against fear and anxiety with their eventualities. A hijacker with a gun commanded passengers not to move. He entered the cockpit. While he was there, a professional comedian got everyone laughing. When the hijacker came back and saw all the people laughing, he concluded they did not take him seriously, lost his nerve, and gave up the hijack!

Herman José, a TV comedian from Lisbon, has great fun making light of political leaders. He aims at only those who themselves see the funny side of life. "Reagan tells jokes. Brezhnev does not. I leave the communists alone because they have no sense of humor." José knows that if people laugh they will survive and go on to victories. Those who cannot laugh have already mapped out their doom.

A doctor said of a friend, "He will never have a breakdown because he has a hair-trigger laugh." Likewise, an insightful leader said of a colleague going through the stress of adjusting to retirement, "He laughs easily so I know he will come through this period of his life O.K."

Humor exposes one's contact with reality. A grip on reality means mental health. Mental health is wholeness.

One of the most interesting experiments in laughter research relates to alcoholism. The South African Brain Research Institute now uses laughing gas, oxygen, and nitrous oxide. They note the reversal of both physical and psychological withdrawal symptoms with a shortening of detoxification periods in 700 subjects who received the new treatment. The success rate is so high that some with expertise in the field of rehabilitation believe the new treatment will become standard.

Current research tells us body chemistry alters with laughter. Use it as a weapon against burnout.

4

Genuine Spirituality

Christ is the indispensable core of effective personal adjustment.

> Lawrence J. Crabb, Jr.,
> "Moving the Couch into the Church"
> *Christianity Today,*
> September 22, 1978

[God's] image is in us, however deeply buried under the debris of our living, and heaven is never beyond the reach of our fingers.

> Thomas Aquinas
> *My Way of Life:*
> *The Summa Simplified for Everyone*
> by Walter Farrell
> and Martin J. Healy

Handling Uncertainties

A chief cause of burnout is inner conflict initiated and generated by indecisiveness. Indecisiveness may come to surface only when teased out by confrontation with life.

The Christian who thought he had his Judeo-Christian morality decided, learns of a church couple living together unmarried. They attend services now and then, do a bit of work for the church, even give money.

Suddenly one feels confused. Have I interpreted the Bible correctly? Were my Christian teachers right? Should I revise my moral beliefs? These questions lead to inner turmoil and mental paralysis.

Stability issues from secure footing. How do we come to grips with uncertainties? How do we keep the channels between us and God open?

Shake loose from the instabilities of the '60s. Grasp the biblical standard. Study, grapple with specific Scripture passages. Deepen your Bible knowledge. A decision to make God's Word your foundation gives you security related to freedom, joy, and health.

Stay close to the Christ of the Gospels. We have four Gospel accounts which tell us about Jesus of Nazareth. Modern scholarship shares a growing respect for these documents (Leslie Badham, *Verdict on Jesus*). The Christ of these dependable documents is our source of personal certainty.

Remind yourself of the validation of gospel truth — the resurrection of our Lord. The resurrection of Jesus was God's way of saying, "What you see in Jesus is really true. This is My method of documentation."

Thomas got that message. So did the early Church. They accepted the resurrection fact. This was the certainty with which Gospel doctrine and Kingdom ethics were proclaimed.

Going On

Expanding spiritual enlargement is a great deterrent to burnout. To increase our scope of understanding in readiness to meet challenges is our aim.

44

How do we do that?

Take the lid off. Sharing is more acceptable now than at any time since the first century. But keeping people at arm's length, externalizing relationships, is easier. The quick and facile answer seldom helps anyone. The shared experience assists both sharer and listener. Loners resist medicine while open people very often get the medicine they need. Contrary to what we might expect, open people find love and acceptance. Loners confront fear and rejection.

Say a resounding "yes" to the inner call. Dag Hammarskjöld's classic response bears repetition: "I don't know Who — or what—put the question, I don't know when it was put. I don't even remember answering. But at some moment I did answer Yes to Someone — or Something — and from that hour I was certain that existence is meaningful and that therefore my life, in self-surrender, had a goal."

This explains a Schweitzer, a Raphael, a Richard Baxter. In medical missions, painting, and preaching, these men got to the center of things. This arrival on center comes with no easy believism, but is the product of honest grappling. It is the essence of health.

Say "yes" every time the call comes. Rossini was criticized because he produced so little in his riper years. He had found the center of things in his magnificent earlier compositions. Riding along on his laurels deprived both himself and the world of even better music.

What makes a person stop growing? Unwillingness to say yes to the repeated urgings. Amy Carmichael rose to the challenge of mission work in India. Later still in India, she heard the call to work with young girls caught in the clutches of prostitution. During the last twenty years of her ministry, though invalided, she ran her girls' home from a bed! Clearly, the way of life lies in saying yes to its strongest and best beckonings.

Who Is Spiritual?

True spirituality is health, the ultimate answer to burnout. What makes the spiritual person? Here are three answers.

Love as a way of life. Dostoyevsky responds through a character, "At some ideas you stand perplexed, especially at the sight of men's sin, uncertain whether to combat it by force or by humble love. Always decide, 'I will combat it by humble love.' If you make up your mind about that once and for all, you can conquer the whole world. Loving humbly is a terrible force: it is the strongest of all things and there is nothing like it."

Love appears forty-seven times in First John, the epistle that tells us love of people is the test of spirituality. Jesus cried out against the eye-for-an-eye way of life and told His followers to relate to persons in the spirit of agape love that expresses consideration selflessly and sacrificially.

Love is the first mark of the truly spiritual person.

Progress. Paul tells Timothy that Christians head for "righteousness, godliness, faith, love, steadfastness, gentleness" (I Tim. 6:11); they don't look back (Luke 9:62; Heb. 6:4); they endure to the end (Matt. 24:12-13; I Tim. 6:12 — contrast v. 9); they run to win the prize (I Cor. 9:24-27). Christians go places and do things; they live not aimlessly but full of desire to arrive at grand destinations.

Spiritual persons grow and go.

Authority earned by submission. The person yielded to God is the spiritual person. The unsurrendered may become the burned-out person without authority over himself or others. Open and humble submission to the Almighty brings one his own authority, and with it His peace, security, and freedom.

Only God can remake us. To try to create a new self, correcting this pattern and mending that relationship, ends only in frustration. Submit to God who will provide freedom, initiative, and creative insight to relate fully to Himself, others, and yourself. In that confident relating lies true authority. It flowers as a result of submission to our only real source of authority, Authority Himself.

Three Flags

F. W. Faber raised warning flags for the person earnest about the spiritual life. Prayer, suffering, and action are the three flags.

Prayer gets at the heart of our religious posture. Freud believed religion escapist, therefore invalid. Many, taking their clue from Sigmund Freud, believe prayer an escape from reality. Prayer that is escapist is sick religion. Jung said much religion is sick, though he came to see real faith essential to health. When prayer operates from a base of genuine belief it is not sick, but the basis of health.

Conceivably someone could burnout from praying. True prayer prevents and heals burnout.

Suffering. Carl Jung, in the 1930s, observed that "about a third of my cases are suffering from no clinically definable neurosis, but from the senselessness and emptiness of their lives. It seems to me that this can well be described as the general neurosis of our time." That statement strikes us as astonishingly current relating to burnout feelings.

The real threat of suffering is a potential for thrusting us into an abyss of meaninglessness. By God's help, we will not fall but rise using daily challenges as steppingstones for creative loving relationships. This is the ground in which seeds of fulfillment will sprout, develop, and flower.

Action looks so terribly good in an activistic society. It may achieve little more than ego-tripping. But when motivation finds its roots in the Word and works of God, the resulting action is divine. Posturing then becomes purposeless, while honestly helping a fellow human being takes on the fullest kind of meaning. The Bible is the story of God's acts; His actions in Christ give us the clue to that helping activity which is born in heaven.

Prayer's Requisite

God is for the desperate, said a man who understands how the Gospel works. God cannot answer requests that say, "I think I can handle this myself," or "If I find resolution to my problem, I can explain it on purely natural grounds." Whatever we discover about intercession and petition comes out of genuine crises like burnout.

To admit a crisis and to face our helplessness opens the door to His grace, and avoids that inner conflict which leads to burnout.

Part of the answer to mounting frustration lies in complete dependence. Sincere application to His will brings regular surrender, which sees prayers answered on a regular basis. Genuine asking brings genuine answering.

Facing crises in solid dependence has a way of demanding something specific from us. Jesus asked persons in need, "What do you want me to do for you?" "Lord, we want our eyes opened." Particularized asking brings particularized answering.

Children figured significantly in Jesus' ministerings because they ask in pristine sincerity. Who can say no to childlike faith? Jesus sees God as Father responding to us with good gifts, not stones for bread or scorpions for eggs. The Father/child relationship says God is Creator and Sustainer, therefore He has at His disposal all I need. He's ready to give when I'm ready to ask.

The hang-up is conditioning that renders us incapable of thinking like little children. That is another way of saying we cannot create faith. The saints declare in absolutely clear terms, "Of course you cannot make yourself a child, nor 'have' faith." That very admission is God's first grip on the knob of our heart's door through which He comes with gift after gift.

And if we suffer such confusion that warped emotions block clear thinking, making a muddle of our wants and needs? This is the reason to bring our desperation to Him to pierce through the fog and restore a balanced outlook.

The psalmist, struggling for childlike faith, cried, "Answer me when I pray. . . ." God did, for the writer of Psalm 4 says triumphantly, "When I was in trouble, you helped me" (v. 1, TEV).

The secret? Dependence despite desperation.

God's Time

One of the keenest causes of suffering and breakdown is forcing oneself to live patiently with a problem. There's a better way than self-compulsion.

I once heard a bishop say he prayed nine years for the solution to a crucial concern. From the glow on his face and the tone in his voice as he preached, it was apparent to everyone that the long course in the School of Prayer was rewarding.

How do we view our long wait?

We see the plight as our best advantage. Help is reserved for the helpless. The long wait makes us feel terribly helpless.

The god who helps those who help themselves is pagan, for the essence of non-biblical religions is do-it-yourself-ism. Sometimes this attitude is demonstrated under the guise of spirituality. Other times it crops up as unabashed humanism in a Christian church. This idea is dead wrong and sooner or later renders one helpless—the condition that can be remedied only by assistance from the true God. A long time may elapse before we come to the point of assistance. Those who have continued through the School of Prayer to commencement witness with valid eloquence.

We see things in realistic perspective. A long wait puts us in touch with bedrock fact. We are compelled to analyze, examine, figure, wrestle, and wonder. The whole process sifts and strains out delusions and downright misconceptions. The resulting perception forces us to take our hands off so God can put His hands on the situation. As long as we think we are in control, we are out of control. We see truth when we live in a surrendered state of mind. Exercising the principle of helpless inadequacy recognizes God's total adequacy. His answer comes in a surprising package at a surprising time.

We thank God that His plan will succeed. Deeply spiritual people testify to the role of praise in patient suffering. Thanks has releasing power, a fact revealed in Scripture and increasingly confirmed by modern brain research. Positive thoughts trigger chemical output which changes outlook. With new sight all kinds of possibilities and creative options offer themselves.

Realizing Dreams

Frustrated dreams cause burnout. Fulfilled dreams bring unsurpassed relief. God favors good dreams.

The first step is to receive God's vision for you. He has power to put great pictures into your mind. He works through sanctified motivations to let us know when we veer from His best will.

The second step is to let God's imagery imprint itself on

your mind. The clue is to resist temptation to fill in the details. Sketch the outline with sufficient boldness to establish a specific goal.

If you sense an urge to pursue a graduate degree for personal growth and professional skills improvement, disregard for the moment courses and research projects. Attend to available options like where to study, what field, or who to study with. Exploration guided by valid prayer will show the way.

A third prayer step is painting your picture big enough to draw the best out of you. The more people who benefit from your dream's fulfillment the more likely that it comes from God. The more demanding the dream, the more it will ask of you. Quality and service are twins. Fulfillment is a happy spinoff of serious personal investment.

Fourth, pray for grace to liberate yourself from comfortable ruts. In youth you dream great dreams, but the wear and tear of life knocks the cutting edges off grand visions. Life may lack the inspiration it once held, even when you have the house and job you worked so long for. Now you need a new vision. Pray for that fresh dream. Without it you perish (Prov. 29:18). An exciting image of your future service to God and man will create the makings of high adventure. In risk lies therapeutic resources.

Pray for the grace to sustain enthusiasm to see your vision come to its most complete and beautiful flowering. Brace yourself with the whole armor of God for coping with challenges that attack your plan. No worthy dream goes uncontested! Pray for grace to receive the new vision, for God is ready to give to those ready to receive.

5

Stress and Distress

. . . most of our tensions and frustrations stem from compulsive needs to act the role of someone we are not. Only he who knows himself can profit by the advice of Matthew Arnold:

"Resolve to be thyself: and know that he
Who finds himself, loses his misery."

Hans Selye, M.D.
The Stress of Life

Come to me, all who labor and are heavy laden, and I will give you rest. Take my yoke upon you, and learn from me; for I am gentle and lowly in heart, and you will find rest for your souls. For my yoke is easy, and my burden is light (Matt. 11:28-30).

Defining Stress

Hans Selye discovered and documented chemical-biologic involvement in stress (adrenal enlargement, increase of corticoids in the blood, weight loss, etc.). Activity triggers matching physiological response. Stress is normal, even needed, to get a job done. Excess stress must be avoided.

Our challenge does not relate to stress but distress. The real challenge lies in discovering: Why does a certain activity bug me, while the same activity does not create unhealthy tension for someone else? We need answers to make living not only bearable, but also vibrant and productive.

The fundamental clue is self-identity. To pretend you are something you are not raises the stress quotient. Depending on the extent of your pretension you can overtax yourself very quickly. Genuine closeness to God facilitates self-identity. Surely our Maker knows us better than we know ourselves.

The follow-up clue is identification of our gifts. Develop skills commensurate with personal talents. Nothing exhausts us faster than doing what we have no talent to do. Sometimes our cultural eagerness to succeed can lead us astray. We migrate toward conspicuous charismatic gifts to find success. Notice calm and collected persons who do not attempt to be something they are not.

Another key is to set life and career goals in line with your abilities. Sort yourself out at the crucial level, then sift activities to match your priorities. You can shape the way you execute assignments to articulate your personality. Tension builds when you try to do things not in your overall goal structure. Distress sets in when you attempt prioritized jobs in a style not your own.

Here, then, is a law of stress and distress: we flourish when we sense work lies within the framework of our goals, talents, and style. When career, goals, or workstyle do not mesh with realistic perceptions of ourselves, distress sets in.

Self-Acceptance

Self-identity comes with difficulty in our Madison Avenue culture. The world, saturated with advertisements bold and subtle, calls us to change. Some changes benefit us, other modifications confuse us.

Researchers tell us that on any single day hundreds of Madison Avenue messages bombard us. We hear urgent suggestions to dress a certain way, use a particular cosmetic to transform our appearance, or go to a hair stylist who will make us appealing. The subtle implication is that we are not all we could or should be. Dissatisfaction sets in, followed by attempts to re-do ourselves. We enjoy satisfaction for a brief period but soon we re-do ourselves all over again.

Advertising philosophy builds on perfectionistic assumptions. Flawless-skinned beauties adorn magazine covers, waxed automobiles appear in show windows, impeccably polished shoes go on display in clothing shops. This does not fit the reality of hard-driving work days. One must learn to pierce perfectionistic conditioning to see himself as a real person. Perfectionism is another cause of burnout.

Simultaneously one must find what he can do well—not perfectly—and proceed to develop and use that gift to the full. Learn to live with yourself as you are, where you are, knowing that everyone is in process. One who lives comfortably with himself or herself knows the secret of avoiding distress. Maturation develops as naturally as blossoms precede tiny green fruit which in turn becomes ripe.

Fruit blossoms initially look alike, but in time the pear, peach, and cherry define themselves. God accepts your age and stage as you are at this moment. Refuse the temptation to think your past worse or better than the present. Refuse to doubt the future. The Christian may believe the next is best.

Believe from the bottom of your feet to the top of your head. Distress will be transformed into hardy, health-generating challenge and godly usefulness.

Reducing Stress by Meditation

Three methods of meditation are typical of some available approaches.

Visualization. Recall any scene from the Gospels. I like to

55

replay the resurrection of Jesus. I see the stone rolling away, Jesus emerging, standing in all His radiance in front of the empty tomb. I look inside. My problems fade and tension diminishes when the victorious Christ pushes out distress. Relaxation quickly sets in.

This visualization technique, employed by ancients and moderns, proves helpful to many contemporaries. The secret lies in the quiet collection of your mind. In that peace the chosen Gospel vignette captures your imagination.

Step-by-step relaxation. Sit in a straight chair, feet flat on the floor, arms dangling. Become perfectly quiet. Now starting with the top of your head moving down relax each part of the body in turn. You may prefer to start with the feet and move up. Slowly, deliberately give yourself time to feel muscle fibers lengthen into inactivity. Having achieved slackening from head to toe, remain in perfect repose. Then open your mind to the fresh coming of Christ. Feel Him enter every fiber of your being. Stay quietly with Him.

This unhurried technique acts as a tranquilizer. It provides a good night's sleep, or new mental agility for a day's work. The secret is to take time to allow relaxation to take hold.

Centering. The Quakers talk about "centering down," the process of cleaning the mind of busyness to give heed to the Inner Voice. Worshiping with Friends in Saffron Walden, England, for some months, I discovered centering takes about twelve minutes. After that quieting period, someone often shared a message from God. Try this in your own private devotion. After ten minutes you will begin to hear God speak.

Saints have utilized the "centering prayer" for generations, achieving similiar results. The focus must be on Jesus Christ. "Lord Jesus Christ, have mercy on me," repeated over and over, can serve as a centering prayer. In both the Quaker and ancient way inner fortitude and deep spirituality have a chance to grow. The personality is pulled together, collected, centered down, and integrated.

While we do not use centering methods primarily to achieve freedom from stress, precisely that comes as a fringe benefit.

Work God's Way

"Let there be no pride or vanity in the work. The work is God's work, the poor are God's poor. Put yourself completely under the influence of Jesus, so that he may think his thoughts in your mind, do his work through your hands, for you will be all-powerful with him to strengthen you." In the same little book *(A Gift for God)*, Mother Teresa of Calcutta goes on to say, "This is always the danger that we may just do the work for the sake of the work. This is where the respect and the love and the devotion come in—that we do it to God, to Christ, and that's why we try to do it as beautifully as possible."

The temptations of the modern secular world can blind us to devoted labor for God. The inflationary spiral worries us, computers reduce persons to numbers, ambition becomes selfish desires. Busyness fronts as success. Temptations with their sneaky infiltrating power can take us unwittingly away from the presence and power of God.

Just at that point stress sets in.

How do we mobilize the Mother Teresa pattern rather than secular stress and distress?

Quietly saturate yourself with the spirit of the living Christ. Find a place isolated from demanding people. One man drives to the ocean and parks. Another enters a cathedral. Still another goes to a retreat center. Select a place where you can isolate yourself successfully. Now silence your mind in the presence of Christ until you make contact. Wait longer, until He occupies every centimeter of your being.

Image Christ working through you. Hear Him talking

through your lips, helping through your hands, walking with your legs, smiling through your face. Visualize people finding help as Jesus uses you. Count on this reality.

Know that Christ lives and breathes in you. Frank C. Laubach achieved this and shared how in *Letters by a Modern Mystic.* The book tells of the stress he experienced working with half a million hostile Moros in the Philippines. He translated frustration into unbelievable achievement. Laubach overcame what could have resulted in burnout.

Diversification

A letter came to me indirectly and anonymously: "I will be working through my contractual year. I don't know what I'll do then. I am really tired of having nonstop responsibilities, so I am taking a leave of absence. I may go on full-time staff at the county social services. I have applied for a similar job in a nearby town, too. I am looking forward to having a job I can go home from."

The frustrated man continues: "The place where I work has been more than generous to me since my arrival. I heartily recommend this place to any one who is excited and fired up, ready to go to it. I just don't have it anymore. I would like to return to school but finances will not permit that. . . . I will appreciate your prayers as I seek God's will." He complains about long working hours adding: "I'm ready for a leisurely nap in a tub of hot water. I think every muscle is crying." (Letter altered for protection of writer.)

This man shows wisdom in seeking a way out of stress. His intense concentration on professional goals over a long period of time has resulted in a lopsided stress quotient. He does not need someone to tell him to quit complaining; he must undergo decentralization or diversification in order to eliminate his obviously heavy stress. How should he proceed?

He must learn to hear his own cry. The inner monitor tries to inform one of the need for diversion. The letter writer did not hear because of busyness that drowned out the messages. His spouse may have tried to help him listen. His symptoms probably included a lack of interest in anything but his job, blaming others for his mistakes, complaining about work load, lack of energy, and a sense of helplessness. This man, whether he continues in his first profession or changes to social services work, must learn his own body language.

He must initiate a program of diversions: swimming, jogging, racquetball, detective books, hobbies, traveling — whatever. He may need to experiment. If one activity does not get his mind off work the irritant becomes one more emotional failure. A pastor suffering hypertension took up stamp collecting at the suggestion of his doctor. He achieved normal blood pressure. Hobbies that function as diversifying agents should not rob one of hours of sleep, be financially profitable, or contain any elements that cheat one of relaxation.

He must develop the habit of diversion before symptoms appear. Traditional cultures like that of the blacks of the South African Veld walk a great deal. They talk to the point of catharsis on a daily basis while enjoying their out-of-doors living room. Those of us who live in urban settings must build something of this relaxed lifestyle into our weekly, if not daily, round.

Retirement and Stress

Anyone facing imminent retirement meets head-on the adjustment challenges others feel to a lesser degree on vacations or weekends. Studies show illness often attacks at leisure times. The days following the Christmas rush are a notable example. The mortality rate of retirees from a major Illinois manufacturing firm is so startling the company is forced to rethink its retirement pattern. Across America retirement frequently leads to meaninglessness, psychosomatic illness, and early death. We call the malady "retirement disease."

When the stress of adjustment makes heavier demands than we can manage, we must find creative ways of looking at retirement.

Accept the challenge. Adjustment does not come easily; face that fact. Do you work at full steam, finding labor at optimum stress level exhilarating? You may be surprised to find yourself addicted to that style. Sleeping in after retirement may prove an idealistic image. You will need to experiment to discover your own balance of rest and action. You must undergo progressive learning to pace yourself in light of your findings.

Discover your own aging rate. The aging process varies from person to person. Enforced retirement for one at peak capacity may indeed kill a man or woman. The mind and body cannot tolerate the enormous distress of meaninglessness. Illness can set in easily with senility, or emotional and sometimes physiological limitations, making happy social contact difficult. The wise retiree discovers productive occupations commensurate with his/her current capacities. Plans, experimentation, and explorations should precede retirement so the line between stopping and starting again is as inconspicuous as possible.

Maintain an open posture. Rigid plans deflate energy especially when they don't materialize. "Open to anything workable," should be our motto. One man with this attitude developed a whole system of ministerial training. Another built a college in the orient, though he never thought of the idea until after retirement. Still another, after a long and successful career in alcohol prevention and rehabilitation work, is teaching in overseas Bible schools. The wise Christian retiree says, "Anything, Lord, that You assign."

Managing Stress

Ask yourself what distress points puncture your skin. The following answers may assist in shaping your own stress management procedures.

Time for tasks. Good managers schedule as much leisure as possible in task achievement. Creativity takes time. When we feel a job could have been done better a residue of heaviness weights the subconscious mind for hours, sometimes days. The cumulative effect of inadequate time and task management may ultimately lead to burnout.

Sagacious scheduling allows for breathers and breaks, laughter and leisure, venting and diverting.

Broken concentration. To do a job a little here and a little there, some now and some later, increases our stress load. Broken concentration means adding time and work for reorientation. Don't hesitate to instruct the secretary to hold calls for an hour or a whole morning. Make clear to family your need for time to do a specific task. We have trouble with this because of our strong religious teaching on availability. The best availability lies in genuine contribution which comes as the result of adequate preparation periods.

Build blocks of time into your work program.

Confrontation. No one likes to face the big animal. Say and do what you must with all speed. Finish the tiger off and make him history so you can get on with the next assignment. Allowing indecision and hesitancy pushes the stress thermometer into the distress zone. Forthright action yields a tremendous sense of achievement. Action's wholesome feeling becomes a major factor in stress release.

Taking yourself too seriously. We ought to subscribe to *Punch,* the marvelous English periodical designed to pull the plug on our terrible seriousness. Certain species of pomposity inevitably lead to unwanted tension. Laughing through the funny papers gives us a better chance of recognizing that mistakes are not leprous.

6

The Therapy of Creativity

A man is never truly himself except when he is actively creating something.

Dorothy Sayers
A Matter of Eternity

Getting Creative

We need to find a creative lifestyle that makes tackling problems stimulating. The best answers to life's challenges reward us by feeding us with new energies. Creative handling of life's work keeps burnout away.

Recognize individual creativity. Search for the tailor-made style that fits only you. Ansel Adam's photographic secret lies in his unique perception of things. He adjusts his camera to pick up what he sees. Rembrandt's genius lay in his special use of light. Beethoven heard themes no one else heard and put them on score paper. How can you utilize originality?

Incorporate creativity into your work. Doing your task imaginatively rather than mechanically makes the difference between liking and putting up with employment. Many dislike their jobs and buy a 'Thank God It's Friday' mentality.

When one's chief motivation is looking forward to the weekend, the five-day work week has lost its power to yield rewards.

A creative spirit can reverse all that to a T.G.I.M. (Thank God It's Monday) mentality that keeps burnout away. Creativity yields excitement then fulfillment and therefore energy. If you cannot be your creative self in your present job, you must look for other employment. But first carefully explore present creative possibilities.

Generate a creative mood. Brainstorm at work to produce an exchange with other creative minds. At home, stir the gray matter by vigorous discussion with the family or relaxants like a hot bath, a deep sleep, or a dig in the garden. Socially, a good meal with friends, a rousing game, even a good laugh can be stimulating. In any setting a habitual posture of enthusiasm keeps the channels open. Willingness to risk fills your subconscious mind with exciting data. Tune your eye and ear to observe life in scope and detail.

Kurt Willinger, an advertisement agency director, says "Everyone has creative ideas at one time or another. The extent and quality depends much on how tuned-in you are to being creative."

Practical Help

Clear your mind for creative action. How? Establish these down-to-earth disciplines.

Start your day. Get up early enough to give yourself a sense of control. Late rising makes you feel like the day controls you. Eat a good breakfast. Take time to get in tune with God, the real source of creativity, and He will show you how to do your work with freshness. Spend time preparing your person and dressing acceptably so that you will feel good about yourself all day. This frees the mind to focus on work.

Allow leisure for your before-work routine so you don't have to rush. These little morning disciplines will reward you by allowing creative juices to flow through the day.

Take care of your body to take care of your mind. Light eating at noon avoids sluggish thinking. Exercise promotes circulation and activates the brain. (Some go to a spa or gym for half an hour of exercise at midday.) Breathing fresh air deeply brings in needed oxygen. Drinking plenty of pure water helps keep the system clean. Avoid smoking. Not only the smoker but also nonsmokers in a polluted room run the risk of cancer problems. A healthy body generates healthy thinking.

Minimize problems by sharing experiences. Talk, write, act—do whatever you must to express yourself. When you've had a rough day at the office don't try to sleep on that pent-up rage lest your rest come to distress and your pulse rate climb. Talk it out or write about it. We need to share good experiences too. All experience needs expression lest it stack up like cord wood until the weight results in cloudy thinking or depression.

Worship regularly. The famous Framingham Study reveals that men who go to church have half as many coronary attacks as men who don't attend public worship. The fellowship of influence and ideas has enormous impact. The presence of God's Spirit means fresh thoughts (sometimes my printed bulletin is filled with notes by the end of the service). Hymn singing clears the mind. Listening to a good sermon brings enthusiasm to life. Talking with friends before and after service means joy and enrichment. The worship experience goes a long way to encourage creative thinking.

Keep your mind ready to create.

Breaking Loose

A major cause of imprisoned feelings is self-imposed limitations. Working in a strict framework fosters a feeling of neurotic security. That false security gets stale as it imprisons.

65

Activate your courage. Break out of your compulsive patterns and rigid habits. The resultant release will prove enormously therapeutic. The windows of creativity may open on to a new and exciting world. Challenges generate enthusiasm for achieving long-range goals.

Notice how quickly your mind clears when you think of fresh ways to prepare a sermon, help a counselee, or build a program. Observe how your associates respond to newness; it becomes contagious while anticipation heightens.

Look at three qualities for breaking loose.

Openness to the Holy Spirit. God's Spirit does not repeat Himself. Document this by looking at spiritual movements. No two are alike, as no two of anything are alike in nature. When you take the easy way of imitating or repeating, you have not listened to God. We grow in our capacity to hear God. As we grow in sensitivity, we come closer to God's exciting innovations. With the execution of each fresh assignment, we grow in wholeness. Nothing fulfills like the knowledge that God's plan has found expression and response.

Courage to innovate. A sturdy independence develops in the innovator. He doesn't always ask, What do people think? He asks often enough to stay in contact with persons, but because "it's always been done like this" is not sufficient reason to continue a pattern of action. What is, and what could be constitute very different perspectives. Courageous thinking brings adventure into one's life. Creative risk may actually bring about revolutionary change. Innovation that creates results in the deepest kind of wholeness.

Living up to your potential. Sloth, one of the seven deadly sins, is not so much laziness as resistance to working up to ability. The nagging realization is that what one could and should be, never will be without substantive changes. That's stress. Peace lies in listening to the Spirit's innovative messages, then collecting courage to do what God says.

Beauty and Creativity

Beauty is God's eloquent witness. Something of this truth shines through Jonathan Edwards' classic assertion that nature is God's best evangelist.

Beauty is far more than a panoramic landscape. It is the shape and perfection of truth. In a sense, truth's order and balance is revealed in peace and harmony.

The experience of beauty brings therapy for our souls. In the presence of the beautiful, healing opens the soul's door with power to penetrate the citadel of the self.

To make beautiful things opens healing doors. Carl Jung sometimes instructed his patients to paint or create something. To create satisfyingly is to feel God and truth impacting our spirits.

Christians create with care that is a dimension of beauty. Sewing a dress, setting a table, doing the gardening, writing an article, producing a tea service at the ceramic shop brings delicious and indescribable fulfillment.

> Its loveliness increases; it will never
> Pass into nothingness; but still will keep
> A bower quiet for us, and a sleep
> Full of sweet dreams, and health, and quiet breathing.

John Keats says more about the restorative power of beauty:

> Some shape of beauty moves away the pall
> From out dark spirits.

Beauty touches God within us. It causes love to flood our minds with a parade of images born of rich experience. Color, light and shadow; sound, sight, and melody; harmony, flow, and contrast; form, shape, and substance say God. They speak inspiration. Beauty, God, and memory team up to ignite creativity within us.

Go to the sea, spend an evening at crafts, read poetry to the family by a winter's fire, walk with your friend in the woods, take up water or oil painting. Learn to give yourself to creative beauty with leisure and whole-heartedness. Watch the puzzle of life come together in meaningful perspective and see the burned-out feeling lift like fog at noon.

Creativity as Medicine

Purpose can keep a human being alive. Purpose with creative possibilities can keep one vibrant, excited, and full of anticipation.

Norman Cousins, in *The Anatomy of an Illness*, discusses two friends, Pablo Casals and Albert Schweitzer. Casals, almost ninety and bent with arthritis, took his medicine from piano and cello. In the morning he played the piano, in the afternoon the cello. Cousins watched stiff fingers become agile and powerful. Casals' back straightened a good deal, his walk lost its shuffle. Ailments yielded to the body's cortisone and adrenaline. Blood pressure increased bringing new vitality to mind and body.

Albert Schweitzer believed that a meaningful job and humor had much to do with keeping illness away. Disease found no hospitality in his body, so illness tended to make its exit quickly. Even after ninety, Dr. Schweitzer worked at hospital rounds and involved himself in strenuous manual labor. He loved to play Bach on the piano at the end of a full day of labor. After playing, Norman Cousins testifies, there was in the old man "no trace of a stoop. Music was his medicine."

Purpose and creativity are twins, the one influencing and shaping the other. Researchers still do not know all that happens when we respond excitedly to stimuli, but evidently vitality and chemistry articulate. Scientists talk about the adrenal system's operation, the pituitary gland, brain impulses, and the endocrine system. Before long the chemistry of creativity will surface as common knowledge.

To open ourselves to stimuli big enough to draw the best out of us, could leave an effect more potent than prescribed medicine. The Holy Spirit, the Spirit of creativity, may well plant in our minds plans whose absorbing presence sparks imaginative endeavor.

Welcome Problems

Problems stimulate us to come up with creative answers. When we find a truly workable answer, the sense of reward is enormous. That sense of reward is a significant way to avoid burnout. How do we develop a relish for creative problem-solving?

Move into neutral. When faced with a problem, you don't know what to do. Rest easily until an answer emerges. Resist the temptation to hurry answers. Relax in the presence of unsolved dilemmas.

Keep flexible. Pascal taught us that the mind solves problems by dialog. The yes-and-no debate goes on inside, continuing until a problem comes to resolution. Do nothing to stop that dialog. Flexibility accepts the dialog's needed range.

Adopt a game spirit. We talk about "playing with ideas." This increases tolerance for ambiguities, diffuses tension, and brings into the decision-making process a sense of fun. Fun is very important for solving problems. Fun releases us creatively. Keep a playful and flexible mood for thought to roam over options and creating new ones.

Maintain a mood of free creativity. Children do. Adults tend to start out enthusiastically, until tension builds clobbering the creative impulse. Children instinctively run for fresh ideas. They don't know "it can't be done" or the ways it can't be done. Herein lies part of the significance of Jesus' words about becoming like a little child. Keep mentally mobile. Children are not tense like the staccato of snare drums, but supple, easy, and fluent like ballet dancers. Fight rigidity like the plague, for it creates a stop in the human spirit. Welcome fresh insight and new information to unplug the mind.

Welcome life's problems; they shake us up. We tend to rid ourselves of ambiguities. Recondition yourself to accept them as opportunities, as sources of stimulation. The cumulative effect of avoiding problems, setting them aside, making hasty decisions, is severe disappointment which may eventually lead to burnout.

Order Out of Chaos

Why do creative persons tolerate ambiguity? Because they know that processing problems, with the attending welter of thoughts, comes eventually to organization. Order follows chaos. But not just any order. A higher order. The emerging organization may have fresh orders that prove better than old ones.

Studies of hippies show that they were not truly creative. Law and creativity are friends, not enemies. Superficial observers mistake the chaos before the order as creativity. Stay with a genuine innovator long enough to see new, workable, efficient structures of connectedness, comprehensions, compression, and relationship.

Ponder creative persons whose scattered yearnings become orderly. The pounding impulses beating in Beethoven's head flowered into the "Fifth Symphony." The shapeless granite hunks facing Michelangelo became sculptures like

"David." The endless static of the early wireless evolved into the pure sound of modern radio.

The profusion of thoughts in planning a board meeting center in an agenda to facilitate goal achievement. The competing ideas that rush to one's mind in the early stages of a writing project eventuate in a meaningful sequence. Flow and overall design are necessary for impact on readers.

This movement from chaos to order is significant for wholeness. Stay in the turmoil very long and you will watch yourself writhe, toss, and wallow. Move resolutely from the struggle to the discovery that the new order will yield a deep sense of satisfaction.

7

God's Gift of Self-Esteem

In every weak person there is a strong person. In every evil person is a good person. In every defeated person is a victorious person. To become aware of this nobility and power within ourselves, is to know and to be able to practice the Art of Living.

Peale and Blanton
Faith Is the Answer

The Beginning Point

From the sin of Adam and Eve to the present, men and women have chafed under self-doubt and physical death. The answer to both is theological. In the next seven meditations we will grapple constructively with self-doubt and God's gift of self-esteem.

Some Christian counselors today see the *Imago Dei* as foundational to help. This means seeing ourselves created in the image of God. When we believe God created us in His image, how can we entertain feelings of self-uncertainty?

Here is the sticky wicket: *Imago Dei* counseling works only if we really believe in God and all He represents. How do we get to the place of firm belief? Perhaps three or four suggestions will assist in the stimulation of your faith.

First, note Bible concepts like *trust, know, believe, assurance.* A basic New Testament assumption is faith, not doubt; confidence, not uncertainty. (See passages like John 3:15; I John 5:14; Luke 1:4; I John 1:1; John 20:31). Certainty is derived from first-hand experience of the living God. God will reveal Himself to those who refuse to hide.

Second, see yourself growing in confidence and faith. Genuine Christians wrestle, probe, face their knowledge gaps, admit perplexities within the godly framework of certainty built on God's promises.

Third, identify with a church whose atmosphere is characterized by New Testament authority. A local church bowing and scraping to secularity cannot give answers; it only creates insecure members. Peter Berger nettles the church for lack of courage that results in "orgies of self-doubt and self-denigration." He calls for a church with guts enough to announce to the world what God says. Berger tells the church to become authoritative. Radical changes in mental outlook in society call for forceful leadership. An authoritative church with a good self-image fosters good self-images.

Finally, in this New Testament church strong in conviction and stance, share yourself and your developing faith. This comes with greater ease in a biblical church than in one weighed down with humanism. The genius of sharing feelings and growing edges is objectification.

Externalization of faith helps us see our thoughts in perspective and provides a way of testing discoveries. It makes us lovable as we migrate toward authenticity. When we're truly loved our self-image gets the best kind of feeding.

Practical Actions

Practice effective disciplines like these to make you feel good about yourself.

Eat good food in a pleasing atmosphere. When you eat more fruits, vegetables, and whole grains than refined preserved foods, you promote health and well-being. If your diet habitually lacks adequate fiber, you know at the back of your mind this is not wholesome, and the specter of disease does not help your self-image. When you sit down to attractively prepared food served in a delightful atmosphere, your mood encourages normal digestion. Aesthetics promote health and a sense of security. Learn the art of eating, for this everyday activity relates to self-concept. When you eat correctly (not in between meals), your weight stays at a medically and socially acceptable level.

Keep energy up. A high fat diet reduces vigor. What we drink also becomes energetics. Insufficient water causes fatigue, excess of Cokes and caffeine drains us, alcohol alters perceptions and causes disease, accidents, and personal embarrassment. Salt used to excess plays havoc with ordinary sources of vitality, notably blood circulation and weight control. Erect posture feeds our subconscious with self-esteem and God-ordained dignity, and spawns health. Adequate sleep (do you require seven or eight hours?) means liveliness too. Review your resources of energy, then program them into your lifestyle. Enthusiastic persons feel good about themselves.

Take advantage of your built-in cathartic system. Nature gave you the means to express yourself. Morton Kelsey advises a daily journal. In the morning record your goals; in the evening write out the day's experiences with fulfilled ambitions and problems solved and unsolved. The released feeling that comes with unloading will lift your spirits. Some achieve the same sense of release by letter writing, others by creation of a novel, and many by talk. A wise couple said they had discovered a four-letter word for psychotherapy: *talk.* Whatever you choose, exercise the gift of catharsis to let loose your true and best self.

How to Get Help

We come into the world with strong egos. Babies have a remarkable and unfettered capacity to rule the roost and make demands. With the passage of time parents, peers, and pressures influence us. This conditioning comes from no malice or forethought, but fears, guilts, and angers pile up to make us fight for ego existence.

One psychiatrist says the most common problem in patients is low self-esteem. He refers them to the New Testament injunction, "You shall love your neighbor as yourself" (Mark 12:31).

True, for the ability to love your neighbor hinges on love of yourself. Love of yourself depends on love of God (Mark 12:30). Fear or hate is a projection of one's low self-esteem and exposes our need for love.

The English talk of getting "thick with God." This is step-number-one in lifting the self-image. Frank Laubach, by nature a timid person, learned to envision himself constantly with Christ. The two of them walked through life together arm in arm. No wonder Dr. Laubach was an overcomer and a winner.

Sometimes simple techniques help—like listing our good points: "I'm a faithful, hard-working spouse; I'm a creative contributor on the local church board; I go out of my way to do kind acts." Anyone can make a list, and even this little exercise brings fresh confidence.

Another method of tackling a shaky ego is to confront the threats that make your ego shake. John Wesley said he always faced an angry mob. The accounts of his victories over rowdyism document the power of eyeball-to-eyeball confrontation. Ralph Waldo Emerson encapsulated this law of life in one sentence: "Do the thing you fear, and the death of fear is certain."

You must face yourself as you are, with your gifts and limitations. To wish to be someone else inevitably erupts in a low level of self-assurance. One of the devil's tricks is to shift our focus on to some impossible goal, a cinch for another but a headache for yourself. God will reveal His assignments and provide matching ability. Following His leadership saves the agony of misspent talents and unnecessary confusion about one's identity.

Perpetually see yourself in a good light. Establish personal and private self-imaging habits that reflect the way God must feel about you. His belief in you will grant self-revelation for growth, vision, energy, creativity, and productivity. St. Paul discovered this for himself. Despite inner wrestling he could say, "I can do all things in Him who strengthens me." History confirms Paul's statement.

Energy, Health, and Self-Image

William James talked about "first-layer" fatigue. We work at a task until we come to a barrier, confess weariness, and often give in. But, said James, if we pierce that layer by force of will and proceed, we find ourselves with new energy, much like a runner getting his second wind on the racetrack.

What makes one person go on and another throw in the sponge? Decision. Positive decision. A positive decision is a vote for yourself.

Our growing discoveries about psychosomatics indicate a first-layer health challenge. See yourself well and you will tend to be well. New information about hormones and glands suggests the flow of beneficial body chemistry when we think positive thoughts. Research indicates that negative thinking— hopelessness, for example, initiates and sustains poor health, and eventually becomes a causal factor in death. Professor Cary Cherniss of the University of Michigan tells us that bored and frustrated people show a blood chemistry different from normally contented persons.

What can we do to encourage hurdling the "first-layer" challenge?

Feed on positive image-builders. See yourself as an energetic disease-free person. The law of homeostasis (when ill or weary the body's natural tendency is to return to its former state of health) known to medical science, puts fresh hope in us. With new zest for wholeness, body chemistry improves and this in turn contributes to normalcy. Health and energy do a lot to foster self-esteem.

Keep busy with your constructive task. Every worthwhile project sooner or later yields rewards. This truth generates energy, health, and self-assurance.

Inferiority feelings are a figment of the imagination. Most negative thoughts are just plain lies. Refuse them. Do it deliberately. Focus on the good which is wholeness and vitality.

Right Living and Self-Image

Holy living lifts the self-image, sin clobbers it. We live by the boomerang effect of doing good and getting good back (Luke 6:38). That feedback nourishes self-esteem.

Notice the biblical marks of right living.

Forgiveness (Matt. 6:14; Eph. 4:32). God honors a forgiving spirit. The knowledge of right relationship with God and others puts us at ease with ourselves.

Right handling of anger (I Tim. 2:8; Prov. 15:18; 29:11; Eph. 4:26; James 1:19). The quickest way to make a fool of oneself is the destructive use of anger. An excellent way to find acceptance is the expression of love and creative problem-solving.

Reconcilability. The classic passage, Matthew 5:21-26, is summarized in the first six words of verse 25: "Make friends quickly with your accuser." Nothing brings inner peace sooner.

To make a friend of an enemy has a tremendous spinoff benefit of making the reconciler feel good about himself.

Sexual integrity (Exod. 20:14; Matt. 5:27-30; I Peter 3:1-7). Sexual lifestyle relates to spirituality and spiritual status helps determine one's self-perspective. Integrity contributes with great force to the construction and maintenance of a strong self-image.

Obedience (II Cor. 10:5; 2:9; I Peter 1:14). One who invests himself in knowing God's will has good reason to feel comfortable. God promises to honor the obedient.

Honor the one true God (Exod. 20:1-7; Deut. 18:9-14). God hates any form of idolatry like money, images, the occult, or self. He respects and rewards all true worship. Poor self-image relates to the false pride that substitutes some thing, idea, or person for God. The one who gives himself to God alone receives God in return. God reveals His presence created in each one of us.

Generosity (Luke 6:38; Prov. 19:17; Matt. 7:1-5; Mark 4:21-25). The giver is blessed while the miser gets nothing in the long run. Generous people don't have to spend time worrying about themselves.

Prayer (James 5:13-18). All the previous marks of right living relate to prayer. To violate any of these is to watch sin impede prayer effectiveness. The relationship of authentic prayer to wholesome self-image is of the highest significance. God gives Himself through prayer for others; His presence has a way of driving out gloomy thoughts about ourselves.

Self-Knowledge

Thomas Merton believed the first step to sanctity is self-knowledge, and that the way to self-awareness is prayer. The serious saints through the ages tell us to cut through the layers of ego and arrive at the center of one's being because God Himself lives there.

How do we strip away fleeting ego concerns, the usual focus of attention, to discover the real self and the God within? This is a fundamental concern.

First we must ask God for *courage*. There is a natural hesitancy about self-exploration; we fear what we may find. That's why we erect elaborate coverings and defenses against self-discovery. Only God can give us grace to explore, and sometimes we need a spiritual guide to help us. Modern seminaries provide guides, soul friends, advisors to assist young men and women over the hurdles of self-finding. By this means today's pastors train to become guides to their parishioners. For all, the process of looking takes courage.

Second, see your social *relationships* as a mirror. We cannot, by raw self-confrontation, really see ourselves. Henry David Thoreau said, "It is as hard to see oneself as to look backwards without turning around." Introspection in isolation yields few results. The word *saints* never appears in the singular in the New Testament, but saints know themselves and the God in them. We learn about ourselves from others.

Third, *love* is the context of self-revelation. Interpersonal relationships can become spontaneous and full of affection; then humor, word, and innuendo are the natural vehicles of information. Without the flow of soul that love brings, fear, hate, and resentment flower, and the process of self-knowledge stops. Study I John 4:13-21.

Finally, *serve* others with all your might. Mother Teresa finds God in Calcutta in the poorest of the poor. There too she finds the meaning of her life. George MacLeod finds God on the Island of Iona where he gives himself to struggling people working in a community setting. Many other illustrations can be given to document fulfilled persons are giving people, self-knowing, and godly. This explains their graciousness.

Be patient. Self-knowledge can never be complete in honest people. But the peace that emerges with growing insight, equilibrium in the presence of others, and serenity-in-depth with God, bring a confidence that frees one to live with abandon.

An Important Clue: Remembering

"We live by our memories." That time-honored proverb reveals a profound biblical secret. In both Old and New Testaments the word *remember* looms large. Many psalms rehearse Israel's victories, and Jesus admonished us to celebrate His supper "in remembrance of me." The Bible teaches us to inspire faith by recalling the turning points of our lives, remembering that God is the Control Agent.

In which direction do we construct our trajectories of thought? Into the black recesses of our Hiroshimas, Vietnams, or into memories bright with moon landings and silicon chips? To decide to live by memories that inspire great possibilities is to nurture a high self-image. Possibility people consistently remember the best and therefore generate success. They foster the beautiful and enrich life's meaning. They also open the door on faith and confidence to bring God close. An impossibility thinker recalls the worst. He cannot live enthusiastically and does not know the joy of the Lord which is strength, ego strength included.

But how do we focus on the good experiences? No one lives without disappointment.

Recall that God and our own natures are for us. Psychologists tell us we tend to forget the bad and remember the good. Self-sympathy encourages negative recall. Reminding ourselves that God is for us is to know that no one can be against us. This fact documented by the life, death, resurrection, and intercession of our Lord, corroborates our own Christian experience.

Now become practical by deliberately talking about good

things at coffee, in the office, at home, or the recreational setting. Today's media journalists believe they usually need to say something negative to capture attention. We have heard so much bad history in our century. We must face the bad and be unafraid to discuss it. Nevertheless, the Christian refuses to live like the 6 o'clock news.

E. Stanley Jones used to say that evil news shocked him, but not for very long, because he knew how history would turn out. The end belongs to God. When our theology is sound and our wills are set we have an unbeatable marriage. To this union come good, true, and beautiful offspring. Each birth marks the advent of new memories to add to the richness of life, thus denying burnout.

8

Physical Fitness

Look to your health; and if you have it, praise God, and value it next to a good conscience; for health is the second blessing that we mortals are capable of; a blessing that money cannot buy.

Izaak Walton
Compleat Angler

There are two places I've never heard of a man having a nervous breakdown. One is in a swimming pool while he's stretching his muscles; the other is in front of a fireplace while he's stretching his soul.

Rear Admiral Lamont Pugh
(former Surgeon General of the U.S. Navy)

Three Antidotes to Stress

Hans Selye's discoveries about biologic reaction to stress suggest that we can fight some stress-related problems with physical weapons. Authorities agree that three instruments work with remarkable efficiency.

Deep relaxation provides opportunity for body processes

to normalize. Perfect quiet brings restoration. This works best for those habituated to regular rest and sleep. Persons presently keyed up beyond peaceful relaxation must patiently recondition themselves. The clue is to sweep the mind of all turmoil. For many, this comes through Christian prayer and meditation (see stress section on meditation techniques). One study suggests persons who sleep five hours or less nightly have nearly twice the premature death rate of those who sleep eight hours.

Physical exercise assists the relaxation process. A good swim may well augur a sound night's rest. Fatigue toxins drain away in vigorous exercise, reducing stress and initiating bodily repose. General body tone increases and strengthens emotional, mental, and biologic defense against physical and psychological diseases. The heart muscle profits from appropriate exercise and arteries stay cleaner. (Your doctor must prescribe an exercise program after age forty or if you have a history of cardiac disease.)

Adequate diet relates to stress and its relief. When artery walls thicken with cholesterol, stress on the heart and circulatory system increases. Causes include beef fat, shellfish, and too many eggs. Sugar and salt add body weight. Overweight taxes the heart and other organs. When these factors join demands of family and work, the result may spell burnout symptoms. Depression increases under these conditions, not to mention a host of common ailments such as respiratory difficulties, arthritic enhancement, and vision impairment.

We have in these three missiles of relaxation, exercise and diet, weaponry tested by both modern science and individual experience.

Signs of Need

Persons who sit a lot run greater physical risk than people at active tasks. Tension and inches have an almost one-to-one relationship. The chest tightens under heavy burdens, blood pressure climbs, the heart suffers damage, and emotions grow abnormal.

The American astronauts discipline their stair climbing, two at a time, as one means of maintaining fitness. If one catches another climbing one step at a time, he's fined money. When lungs supply sufficient oxygen to heart and brain, one handles stress without breathlessness, pounding pulse, or lightheadedness.

Normal weight keeps us in good physical condition. Modern medical research, as well as common sense, tells us that each excessive pound of fat means more work for the heart. This risk can be eliminated by discipline and guidance. The tricky thing about weight is the power to multiply. An average of two pounds added yearly can mean twenty excess pounds in ten years, forty in twenty years, eighty in forty years. Little by little heaviness sneaks up.

Resting pulse beats of eighty or under generally mean one lives inside the margin of safety. Overweight plus a sedentary life often produces a rate outside the safety zone. In such cases, any number of diseases may invade, especially coronary ones. Dr. Laurence E. Morehouse, Director of the Human Performance Laboratory, University of California, Los Angeles, says: "The mortality rate for men and women with pulse rates over 92 is four times greater than for those with pulse rates less than 67." He finds the average rate in men 72-76. Professor Morehouse also speaks to the person with an irregular heartbeat, making clear that too is a warning sign. The doctor must evaluate both accelerated and jumpy heartbeats.

Headaches, stress, and high blood pressure often go together. Year upon year of those symptoms can issue in stroke, kidney failure, or other problems. For many, attitude is the most significant therapy. Diet and a proper rest pattern also figure in the cure. Stabilizing drugs and exercise can supply still further assistance, as your doctor will tell you.

How to Help Yourself

Try to evaluate your situation objectively. Consider eating and drinking habits. Candies, soft drinks (really saturated sugar), and too much pasta can do such things as add weight and increase sluggishness. One study shows 250 milligrams of caffeine a day (2½ cups of coffee) generally do not hurt humans, but consumption of four or more cups increases risk of heart attack, nervous disorders, and high blood pressure.

Smoking half a pack per day ups the risk of death by heart attack some 60 percent, a full pack by 110 percent. We can argue that so and so smoked a pipe and lived to ninety-three, but such instances appear more anecdotal than scientific.

The relation between muscle tone and the condition of the heart is well known. Paul Dudley White says firm thighs mean a good heart, and he examines thigh tone before doing surgery. An exercise program, especially walking, can keep muscles in shape.

Exercise will help keep us relaxed, do away with midday fatigue, bring us home bright and energetic at the close of the day.

Your doctor will tell you all this and more. You need to hear it from him to give urgency to motivation. Every adult past forty should go for an annual checkup.

Persons who don't have time to attend to fitness may not have much time at all. Joe died in his fifties. He gave little heed to dieting and exercise, and never conquered tobacco. Arteries clogged, surgery succeeded in extending his life only a few months.

The price of vitality is discipline. The kind Dick put into practice. One cardiac arrest after another could not deter his determination to get well. Slowly, surely he developed his body by jogging and diet, strengthened his mind by reading, and organized his observations into a vast and eminently useful filing system. He grew close to God by prayer and meditation. Today he lives a normal, productive, and very busy life as a pastor.

Benefits of Weight Control

Stress is the chief health challenge in contemporary America and the Western countries. Overeating is a response to stress. Over half the adult population in the U.S. weigh more than standards indicated in traditional life insurance charts.

Weight problems often relate to childhood. Heavy parents feed their children too much, and studies show they even overfeed pets. Fat cells accumulate in the early years. Currently, modern medical science has no way to reserve hypercellular accumulation. Poor food management often starts not in childhood but at about twenty-five years of age. This is the time one begins to sit more and eat richer foods. Stress begins to translate into distress.

The classic formula for calculating correct weight for women works like this: a height of five feet calls for 95 pounds; add five pounds for each inch—so a 5'5" female should weigh 120 pounds. Weight for males figures on the same principle, but starting at 10 pounds heavier (105 pounds for a five-foot man)—thus, at six feet ideal weight is 165. Recent research suggests more liberal base figures. There are, of course, other slight variances (age is not one of them for optimal health), but the classic formula indicates a norm for longer and more fulfilled living.

The penalty for excess weight includes nearly everything: money (considerable amounts over the long haul), emotions (sluggishness, depression), aggravated medical problems (diabetes, arthritis), initiation or near-initiation of physical problems (cardiac arrest, stroke).

In contrast, the tremendous benefits of normal weight seem without number. Surgery is far less dangerous due to greater pulmonary reserve, lower incidence of anesthetic complications, less fat tissue for the surgeon to contend with. When one goes for an annual checkup the doctor experiences less difficulty in abdominal examination (to locate organ enlargement, tumors). Clinical procedures come with greater ease in persons of normal size. The psychological rewards include acceptance by society. Sheer physical energy is the greatest benefit.

Weight control reduces frustration and therefore helps minimize the possibility of burnout.

Taste for Exercise

Exercise has its own attractions and we easily develop a taste for it. Research indicates some develop addiction to jogging! Exercise can sometimes defeat pain, sickness, or inertia.

What makes physical exercise so attractive?

Activity and use. After years of intensive exercise-physiology research, we have abundant documentation for what man intuited. Whatever is used is kept in running order. Arm muscles cannot atrophy when one lifts weights, legs cannot go limp if one walks. Just as the mind sharpens with use, the body tones up with exercise. For all-round health and well-being, few things beat exercise. Positive documentation shows that exercise is one method for the control of cholesterol.

Thought and exercise. If sluggishness can result from overeating and inactivity, alertness can increase through moderation and exercise. Take a run and a shower before a particularly taxing meeting. You will document for yourself the relation between physical fitness and mental agility. Oxygen gets to the brain, circulation improves, and a general tenor of well-being creates a mood of confidence and calm.

Working out and appetite. Craving for food diminishes, often vanishes, with a good run or a fast game of racquetball. Physiological changes account for this phenomenon. Emotions suggest eating as a diversion from the heavy day at the office. However, changing into a sweatsuit and tennis shoes for physical exertion means refreshment and the ability to wait for supper.

Calories and weight control. Walking burns calories at the rate of five per minute, swimming at eleven each sixty seconds, and running at a rate of nineteen. A thirty-minute swim would burn up the calories in a piece of pie. While vigorous activity assists in the elimination of fat, controlled food intake remains the chief way to stabilize weight.

Emotions and the out-of-doors. Inside activities like running laps in the gymnasium have their place, but fresh air and scenery have a way of releasing the mind to newness and injecting fresh stimulation. The effect may be the sense of starting all over again, for problems reduce to size, fatigue goes, mental processes unclog; all this equals a measure of renewal. A regular exercise regimen can have cumulative effects, staving off burnout syndrome and building a defense against the onslaughts of daily life.

Nutrition

The central challenge of the budding science of nutrition is to furnish food and food supplements sufficient for adequate energy without accumulation of harmful fatty deposits. Here are some current guidelines:

Energy and health levels can come up with improved nutrition. Colds and flu occur less frequently to those who give attention to what they ingest. Fatigue, even aging, can modify under programmed nutrition. Dr. Michael Colgan, recent researcher at Rockefeller University, New York, says, "My strength has increased more than one hundred percent in the last seven years. And I've changed from a complete skeptic about vitamins to one completely convinced." (See *Omni*,

Vol. 4, No. 7 for elaboration on Colgan's work and vitamin science data.)

The body requires six elements: water, vitamins, minerals, carbohydrates, fat, and protein. Water facilitates organ function, plays a role in turning food into energy, and occupies 60 percent of body mass . . . The purer the water we drink, the better. Carbohydrates, in some grains, sugars, and starches, give us energy but must be eaten in moderation. Fats must be consumed even more cautiously. They yield nine calories per gram of food as compared with four calories per carbohydrate gram. Protein, like carbohydrates, yields four calories per gram and serves as a body builder and defender against illnesses. Food charts, available from qualified dieticians, provide guidance for balanced intake. (See *The Un-diet* by Robert J. dePuis, M.D. for expanded information.)

Specific attention to vitamin/mineral intake pays dividends. The vitamin/mineral revolution can revolutionize us. Casmir Funk, Polish biochemist, discovered the first vitamin in 1911. Vigorous research continues and currently documents nearly half a hundred components demanded by the body. Generally the body cannot manufacture its own vitamins. Vitamins are essential for cell maintenance, but supplements do not always come up to advertisement claims.

Our challenge is to get enough quality vitamins and minerals for energy heightening. That kind of information will likely come from competent professional guidance. One sound source is Dr. Marshall Ringsdorf, professor in the Department of Oral Medicine, University of Alabama in Birmingham. (He graciously answers all mail inquiries.)

Minimize animal/dairy fats (saturated) in favor of vegetable and corn oils (unsaturated). This assists in moderating collections of fat and cholesterol. Beef appears to be a chief villain. Many people are told to avoid organ meats such as liver and heart, as well as marbled cuts. Fish, chicken, and turkey serve as good substitutes for beef, eggs, and yellow cheese. For long-range health and improved mileage, the challenge is to find foods low in calories with elevated nutrients.

Nutrition can be programmed for vital, productive living. One researcher discovered in fast-food portions additives that included pesticides and defoliants. Add to internally taken toxins those that attack from the air and environment (pollutants, noise, speed) and one begins to sense the need for combatants. We have research to show the lowering of immunological efficiency (50 percent in some studies) in the presence of generalized stress. Defenses can be erected through nutritional controls and vitamin intake.

Nutrition is a normalizing factor. The results of careful nutrition show troubled persons normalizing physical, mental, and emotional behaviors. Injury and infection shrink, absenteeism diminishes. Depression lifts. One psychiatrist says 20 percent of psychotics can normalize with balanced diet (see "Nutritional Psychosis," *Omni*, Vol. 4, No. 8). The whole defense system strengthens with balanced eating and by ingesting vitamins and minerals.

Conclusions demonstrate that what we eat and drink relate to what we are emotionally and physically. We must face the call to reorientation, reconditioning, and personal discipline as ways to fight burnout fatigue.

9
Time

I take on too much because there are so many fun things to do: teaching, consultations, video projects —creative things that I love to do, but don't really need to do. A calendar gets full very fast.

"Time for Things that Matter,"
Ed Dayton, *Leadership*,
Spring 1982

Stewardship of Time

Research I conducted on fitness included the spectrum of physical exercise, sleep, vacation, study, hobbies, devotional experience, and sharing groups. My aim was to discern the level of fitness in the clergy. Research subjects included American whites and blacks, South African whites and blacks, Britishers, persons from many denominations, the moderately educated and those with advanced degrees, old, young, and middle-aged ministers. What I did not fully anticipate was facts about the way ministers use their time.

I knew that some live carelessly. What I did not know was that virtually all studied have areas of their lives which are under no discipline of time. Even vacations and rest for renewal surfaced uncertainly. I suspect a major reason lies in the goal—conflicted nature of church work. We work to achieve such wide diversification that we sometimes suffer a paralysis in knowing where to spend our time. Another reason possibly relates to the personal freedom clergy have after theological training. Another cause lies in the pastor's availability, which means people often take advantage of his time.

What concerns me is the inevitable frustration due to unfulfillment. My completed research indicates that clergyman after clergyman does not set aside adequate time for sermon preparation, prayer, Bible reading, family holidays, and personal recreation. Feelings aroused by unproductiveness spell fatigue and discouragement. Here lies a major reason ministers burn out and leave the ministry. I saw on the returned survey sheets many attempts to cover up feelings of exaggerated guilt, posturing, and excuse-making.

An answer lies in prayerful decisions to correct the situation. Charlie Shedd's *Time for All Things*, builds on the principle that time management is a theological matter. This truth is a spiritual challenge. We shall be called to account for use of time resources (Matt. 25:1-13; cf. Eph. 5:16).

The first step is decision in the presence of God. Step two is to see priorities of God first, family next, work third. This is the larger framework in which God calls us to operate. Within this structure, we exercise our gifts and the disciplines of time.

By designing our days under God we can avoid exercises in futility. Then we will find ourselves making time for achieving salient goals. What can loom more satisfying to Western man than just that?

Another Look at Priorities

God, family, work—this is a sound priority perspective. Recently I heard of another perspective. Kathleen and I received an invitation to attend a theological school commencement at which the Archbishop of Canterbury would give out diplomas and address the graduates. We were to stay for lunch and the dedication of a new student facility.

The new building was a student commons primarily for recreation. The archbishop stated that a recreational center carries importance second only to the chapel in a theological college. He explained himself in terms of a threefold priority scheme of prayer, rest, and work. "I wish I had followed that priority program better," said the middle-aged prelate. He fervently hoped the divinity students and graduates would accept it.

Often our conditioning dictates guilt if we do not fill every minute with "worthwhile" work. The falsity of this premise documents easily: simply list the unnecessary work activities in which you engage.

Peter Drucker's incisive comments published in *Leadership* (Spring 1982) refers to Harry Hopkins, President Roosevelt's confidential advisor in World War II. A sick and dying man, Mr. Hopkins could work but a few hours daily, requiring him to identify only the most crucial concerns. The upshot? Hopkins "accomplished more than anyone else in wartime Washington."

God calls us to free our minds of the myth of indispensibility. Ed Dayton (*Leadership*, Spring 1982) believed, We're afraid something will "slip through the cracks." He found a psychological solution. "I asked myself, 'What happens when I'm off camping in the woods for three weeks? The world somehow gets along without me. . . . So you miss one out of ten important articles. So what?' "

So then, maybe the prayer-rest-work priority can come to reality. That would go a long way toward avoiding burnout.

A Stratagem for Managing Time

The pastor kneels at the altar of his church sanctuary each morning. During the thirty-minute period his note pad fills with God's assignments for the day. Quality control means good use of time. Without controls, time wastes like water down the kitchen sink.

God has ways of telling us what to do and what to eliminate. Robert Louis Stevenson observed that the genius of art lies in omission. Time management is an art. No work comes to its intended fulfillment without the right (godly) use of time.

What astonishes us about "Be still, and know that I am God" (Ps. 46:10) is the context of war (v. 9). Evidently the psalmist had so oriented himself to the voice of God with the sense of His presence that he could quiet himself in the thickest battle.

Silence is the sealed recording studio where we hear God. He speaks after the closed door drowns all noise. Then, the messages come, to surprise and bless. The best message is God Himself who provides strength and ingenuity to use time to maximal benefit.

John Greenleaf Whittier writes "the silence of eternity" in verse three of his hymn, "Dear Lord and Father of Mankind." Verses five and six spell out "the silence" and reveal victory over hassle and time-fighting.

> Drop Thy still dews of quietness
>   Till all our strivings cease:
> Take from our souls the strain and stress,
> And let our ordered lives confess
>   The beauty of Thy peace.
>
> Breathe through the hearts of our desire
>   Thy coolness and Thy balm;
> Let sense be dumb—let flesh retire;
> Speak through the earthquake, wind, and fire,
>   O still small voice of calm!

The art of time management is the art of silence. No contemporary challenge looms more urgently than the construction of resources of quiet. Someone said our culture has "almost outlawed silence."

96

We must develop resources by which we rid ourselves of push. In quiet we lop off distractions ridding ourselves of obsessions until the ear expands to full listening range. Thirty minutes a day over the years will result in a resource center complete with divinely designed data bank and retrieval system.

Hurry Is the Devil

"Hurry is not of the devil," said a wise man, "hurry is the devil."

Ponder the implications of rushing through a task only to live with the frustration of mistakes. We vary in our ability to orient. Deliberate minds are often more creative. Imaginative answers require seeing all the way around a matter. Memory and concentration relate to one another bringing fulfillment.

A fundamental law of life emphasizes: don't push. Beating the clock means push with broken concentration. Doing a task to get it over with, spells push. Can anyone imagine the birds or jungle animals racing time to stack up brownie points?

Meaning issues from doing tasks well. This is the just consequence of relating openly, humbly, and therefore unhurriedly, to people. Forcing persons to decisions before they are ready creates rebellion and withdrawal. God has intended time as the instrument of healthy interpersonal relationships.

We must resist hurry. The architecture, interior atmosphere, and traffic patterns at fast-food restaurants have been expertly designed to keep everyone moving. Fast food is a paradigm of our age. To see the calculated dynamics helps us stay current with the subtle manipulations of our restless world.

Practical suggestions? (1) Prepare a sack lunch to eat in

the park. No law commands us to go through the day breath-lessly. (2) Take a realistic look at your traffic pattern. A den-tist lies down in his office for a thirty-minute nap at 5 P.M., and arrives home as soon as if he had left the office at rush hour. (3) Find a way to defuse the mad rush inside. An air-craft manufacturing executive dictates memos for the next day on his way home from the office. He is able to meet wife and family with a clear mind and serene spirit.

Take time to personalize your plans to defeat "push" and "hurry."

Time and Incentive

Time without incentives bores us. With motivation, time fills with substantive activity that gives a sense of achievement.

Psychology Today polled 23,000 people to discover what modern workers want in a job. These six priorities were listed: (1) increase self-esteem, (2) accomplish something worthwhile, (3) learn something new, (4) develop skills and abilities, (5) have freedom on the job, (6) do what one does best. Of the eighteen items rated, job security came eleventh, pay twelfth, fringe benefits sixteenth.

Time, in America especially and in the Western world generally, is a valuable commodity. It is the carrier of mean-ing, not merely the instrument for making money. If time fills with inflexible routine, robbing us of personal initiative, meaninglessness sets in. Boredom means work no longer delights the worker.

Some companies have tried flextime, a way employees can put in their eight hours between seven A.M. to six P.M. An established period in the heart of the day (something like ten A.M. to three P.M.) can help insure "care of the store." Some organizations permit four ten-hour days. These kinds of flexibility may facilitate the priorities listed above.

One can inquire of the employer about the feasibility of flextime. Persons in management positions can map out time schemes with increasing proficiency (see Spring 1982 issue of *Leadership*). When some misuse flexibility, problems multiply in terms of product quality and quantity. Used to good advantage, flextime can introduce inspiration, upping work level and personal satisfaction. (Data on the six opportunities study and flextime from Beverly A. Potter, *Beating Job Burnout*.)

Why Do I Keep So Busy?

Start with the truth about yourself. If you are projecting a childhood movie of your mother's idea of you, you can expect to live a very busy double life. Strength also drains away when you live with some unsurrendered problem.

A work of the Spirit is cleansing of self to make us transparent. Then we do not need to keep overbusy for fulfillment. We can focus our efforts to get God's assignments done.

Sensitivity to human needs holds another answer. Christians called to help hurting persons fervently yearn to alleviate suffering. We try to assist too many people. We need to learn to say "No" as well as "Yes" prioritized by consideration of our special talents.

Persons in the helping professions have pressures to do. We must question whether our "availability conditioning" needs revision. Do guilt feelings arise from a truly biblical authority base? Am I compensating for inferiority feelings? Am I trying to build a power block at my place of work? Am I frenetically attempting to get more from my people than they can give? Am I working to live up to some societal or community standard? Am I compensating for or covering up vocational dissatisfaction? Am I seeking to escape failure by an overfull calendar?

When we set aside time to ask crucial questions, we must quiet ourselves to listen to His answers within a leisurely time frame. Sound answers can save you from burnout.

Rhythms

William L. Shirer, revered American writer in his seventies, goes to work at 9 or 9:15 each morning. He used to write straight through to 3 P.M. "Now I find I'm starting to look at the clock about a quarter to two and I write from four-and-a-half to five-and-a-half hours, and that's all I can do. I've had it for the day." Then he takes lunch and a brief rest, followed by gardening or sailing. In the concert season he attends a recital to satisfy his insatiable love of classical music. He lives in Lenox, Massachusetts near Tanglewood, summer home of the Boston symphony.

Shirer has learned when to work and when to quit. He knows how to change his rhythms of labor and recreation as he grows older.

The current Archbishop of Canterbury, Robert Runcie, keeps pigs. He says he could never boast about being a good archbishop, but could say he's an excellent pig keeper. This good man knows who he is in the balance of labor and hobby, sobriety and humor, humility and ego.

How do we find our individual rhythms? *Rest.* Notice the work/rest motif in Scripture. God rested on the seventh day after creation. Jesus often went away, sometimes with His disciples, sometimes alone. The Book of Hebrews instructs us to strive for and plan rest. Through the Bible we have references to rest and refreshment (e.g., Gen. 8:9; Exod.

23:10-11; Lev. 26:34-35; Isa. 30:15; Matt. 11:28-29; Heb. 3:7 – 4:13). Written in His Word is the rhythm of work and rest.

Experiment. Learn who you are. Some thrive on long, nonstop work hours. Michael Cassidy, founder of Africa Enterprise, can begin early in the morning and go to midnight. Few can do that. Make your own discoveries. When work makes you lethargic, change, find a new set of stimuli, take a break.

Observe the needs of others. A person's challenge relates not so much to oneself as to family and employees. Their needs too must be met in relaxed coffee klatches, picnics by the sea, routines shared. Balance or rhythm must be worked at conscientiously.

10

Family

A husband may beat his wife, but she will love him; he may commit adultery, but she still loves him; but if he ignores her with silence, she will leave him.

Anon.

Family Support

The landmark study of 7000 survivors in the *American Journal of Epidemiology* demonstrated that those who could depend on strong family ties had a much better chance of recovery from cancer and cardiac diseases. Sufferers living with poor family support systems show a vivid increase in the death rate.

Loving affirmation in our families may literally be the difference between life and death. Psychosomatic studies demonstrate the clear relation between depression and physical illness. After trauma depression may set in, then comes disease, and even death may follow.

Support is not over-solicitous attention to one another. It

is the ministry of presence. Like the ministry of Jim and Doris, who have spent their lives "being there" with letters, phone calls, money, anything we mean by personal attention. They travel the earth, even at 80, to be with their family and friends. Flattering people would not suit their real ministry.

How do they minister? They *listen*. Jim and Doris really don't talk much, but they always have time to lend an ear. "Listening is silent love," the most eloquent kind of therapy and support. It is a profound expression of selflessness, and goes a long way toward relieving burnout.

They *accept people just as they are*. When people come across full of self-pity, bitterness, and jealousy, never mind—accept them. For a family member to listen with full acceptance gives the joy that creates hope. Hope is medicine.

Jim and Doris *refuse to pamper* people. They prod gently, subtly, patiently, but firmly. They never scold, that serves only to deepen problems and add guilt feelings. They bring people to a point of clear thinking that opens windows to reality and a way out.

Jim and Doris let you know they are on your side. They have the spirit of affirmation; they give family support.

Forgiveness

We can thank God for the current movement to expose abuse of wife, child, or aged person. Some of the worst abuses are those against children: sexually, verbally, or physically. Damage is primarily to emotions that make adult self-identity and self-worth elusive. At maturation the alert victim sees clearly the damage done by parents or siblings, and anger erupts.

Forgiveness is God's provision for handling anger. Family

members who forgive one another stay together happily. As a minister attempting to help hurting families for over three decades, I have seen very few problems unrelated to the angry, unforgiving spirit.

A wife who was involved in an affair has the ugly festering thing to live with. She fears her husband will refuse forgiveness if he hears what happened.

Sometimes a father who has abused his young son tries to be reconciled by doing favors rather than by asking forgiveness. The best gift to give his grown son is honest reconciliation to relieve them both.

When parents will not talk out abuses of past years, children must learn to forgive by God's grace. The lessons learned may be put into use in rearing their own children.

How do we forgive those who have hurt us? The Bible instructs us to love the people who inflicted pain (I Peter 3:9; Rom. 12:14; Matt. 5:44; Prov. 25:21). Giving cool water to those who harmed us does not generate enthusiasm. Forgiveness is humanly impossible because with great power and tenacity resentments grip the wounded soul.

Only God grants grace to take the first step toward love so that we develop the capacity for forgiveness. God does even more by giving a sense of understanding and compassion for the offenders. He loosens the tenacious grip of resentment and resolves conflicts to bring the *shalom* of healing. His *shalom* can be profound healing from burnout.

Love

Gut-level affection that releases family members to relationship and fulfillment is more difficult to develop and maintain than sentimental love.

Practical, gut-level love is key in these illustrations: a school boy whose preoccupation with home problems robs him of concentration, a mother whose psychosomatic illness resists treatment because family love bridges need repair, a husband who cannot function competently at work because his wife is cold and distant.

An exciting movement in contemporary health care is "holistic medicine." For example, there is a clinic where the doctor in charge listens to the patient's "whole" story. Family members participate to clear the air of tensions and misunderstandings. The doctor patiently opens channels to restore free-flowing love. He knows harbored resentments can cause major disease; he knows love that cancels resentments is the therapy to make possible success of other therapies.

Experts tell us that traditional medical practice of drug and surgical remedies may not meet the complete needs of a patient. Primary therapy must come from the family itself. This is the therapy called love.

Love therapy begins with genuine friendship, the kind Henry David Thoreau talked about: "The language of friendship is not words, but meanings. It is an intelligence above language." When individuals in a family are taken for granted, they cease to be friends. When we relate to one another with respect and attention, self-images climb. Disease can reverse into health when a sense of acceptance pervades our subconscious minds and comes to outward expression.

"The greatest happiness of life," said Victor Hugo, "is the conviction that we are loved, loved for ourselves, or rather loved in spite of ourselves." Modern psychotherapy says the same when it announces that love has power to cure virtually every disorder, burnout included.

Independence

Julius Fast observes in *Body Language*, that all creatures map out their own space. They will fight to earn or keep it.

"This is my territory" is a hallmark of God's creations. Physical space symbolizes and makes tangible psychological space, space essential for independent movement.

Overcautious parents ("Why can't you act like your father?") thwart the normal process of individuation. Rebellion in teen years results from urges to be one's own person in one's own space. A good deal of frustration comes from feeling imprisoned in another's territory. Breaking out of childhood can take either socially acceptable or anti-social expression. The realization of full personhood does not occur without independent existence.

We must give our children kindly guidance built on God's Word. We dare not dominate them for later conflicting emotions will thrust them into mental anguish. Husbands and wives must respect each other's own personality. Chauvinism on the part of either man or woman crushes the human spirit. One aim of marriage is to encourage fulfillment of each. Our assignment is to let God be God in one another. And when that biblical freedom exists, the natural flow of life we call happiness has opportunity to come to blossom.

"Letting go and letting God" may not come easily for highly motivated parents or spouses. We want perfection, now! God wants to infuse us with grace to shape our aspirations with holy realism. This tempers our personal approaches to achievement with divine graciousness. He wants to develop in us a style that invites spontaneity, the respect of "live and let live."

St. Paul says that "where the Spirit of the Lord is, there is freedom" (II Cor. 3:17). When you invite His Spirit into your home to create an atmosphere where individuals have space, don't be discouraged by your own rough edges. Remember we're all in process. The very next verse (18) announces the good news that we "are being changed into his likeness from one degree of glory to another; for this comes from the Lord who is the Spirit."

A Sense of Place

Lawrence Durrell, a descriptive writer, learned to identify places so completely that his portrayals are luminescent paintings ready to hang in a national museum of art. His writing on Egypt—Alexandria, the Nile, Aswan—(*The Alexandria Quartet*) documents his unusual talent. When asked how he achieves his intimate descriptions, he comments on the capacity to concentrate. Close your eyes, he counsels, then see the fullness of your surroundings. Fuzzy writing issues from inaccurate and incomplete visualization. One must paint the picture in mental detail before transferring it to paper.

Creating the spirit of place for each member of our family requires a parallel investment of thought and action. Close your eyes. See, in detail, the personal needs of your partner or child. Study to meet those perceived needs in the twin contexts of daily living and personality structures. When mom bakes dad's favorite apple pie and sets it on the table with the best of cheeses, father feels "at home." So does mother. Both have found a piece of "place."

Paul Tournier believes "place" essential to good counseling. Two chairs in front of the well-laid fire create "at home-ness" that is itself part of therapy. Natural healing takes place where comfort-in-depth enters the soul. The place called home partakes of heaven supplying the consolation required by all normal human beings.

To make home a retreat where one experiences refurbishing of mind and spirit, makes possible facing the work-a-day world with its burnout threats. To invest ourselves knowingly, gently, firmly, gives rise to that fuller acceptance we define as "place." Freshly cut roses on the coffee table, silver candlesticks at dinner, the tender touch of a hand during the late late show, paint on life's canvas the colors that make one feel fully trusted.

The freedom to trust and to be trusted creates the sense

of "place." The little amenities of life document the reality of that profoundly needed experience.

Life's Laboratory

The family is a little laboratory for learning how life works. In the family we learn the secret essence of living.

How do we insure a context of learning in families?

Live together. In Russia one in three marriages ends the first year. Abortion is so common that some women have half a dozen abortions, some as many as eighteen (London *Times*, July 17, 1982.) The Russian government currently tries to get women out of factories and back home. Why? The best education is in the home. Avoiding responsibilities by divorce, abortion, or unreasonable work outside the home reduces the scope and range of family learning.

Live together in love. Love allows everyone to be him/her self. Such a circle of kith and kin does not construct a utopia where only perfect people live; good families allow one another to make mistakes and get rewards for worthy accomplishment, and learn from these experiences. The confidence generated in such an atmosphere is premium fuel providing energy to participate in life with enthusiasm.

Live together in fun. Wholesome families learn the genius of variety and balance. We cannot work all the time; games have their place too. So does teasing which gently exposes our inconsistencies. Overseriousness, like artifice, results in loss of perspective.

Live together in a real world. Family life teaches realistic expectations. To reach too high means disappointment; to bend too low results in boredom. Family dialog assists in discovering that middle ground which is realism, and helps us learn that life is not made of people who smile beautifully all the time, smell like a flower garden, and make money effortlessly. A study of Harvard graduates summarizes their consensus: "It's a lot harder out there than we were given to believe in university." Sound family units project the nature of the real world.

Live together in readiness to help one another cope. When one member of the family comes home absolutely exhausted, sensitive families feel the rejection he has received. When one divorces himself from active involvement, know that he has been disappointed. When one turns critical, even sarcastic, his enthusiasm has been dampened by resistance or attack. In each example the drained, detached, or cynical one faces a cul-de-sac. Empathetic families open discussion facilitating resolution.

The laboratory training a family can give prepares people for the harsh world, sends young people off to school, work, or marriage with coping instruments. No family prepares each one thoroughly against some burnout. But an empathetic family can provide the timbers that go into building strong emotional constructions.

Privacy

Today's emphasis on openness is good and bad. Learning to share strain and stress is good; however, we can never force privacy to yield its needed secrets. Secrets must be discovered at their own speed. The whispered delights before Christmas, birthdays, Father's and Mother's Day, anniversaries, and Valentine's Day symbolize our basic need for secrets.

Secrets have a wholesome privacy that says we belong to ourselves. Family members who pry, create overdependency or inflict hurt. Employers who must know everything create servile employees. Drive vanishes when personhood is threatened.

Burnout takes place when the rewards derived from personal initiative vanish. When what I do only serves someone else's ends, fulfillment evades me. I must be allowed freedom to create my own excitement with the liberty to share when I'm ready.

When Terence Conran, celebrated designer, saw himself becoming rich he determined to help his staff make money too. His employees receive shares with their salaries. If workers leave the organization their earned shares go with them. The whole program declares Conran's belief in people as persons.

When corporations and families succeed in cultivating personhood, burnout is defeated. The positive feedback acts as fuel to create health, energy, ideas, and achievements. Enthusiasm comes from the sense that "I" can do important things. This private "I," when kept intact, functions very well.

Every family should read Paul Tournier's *Secrets*. The little book reveals the need of children to have secrets that develop their personhood. Maturity, Tournier says, lies in the freedom to keep and share secrets. He believes his own success as a counselor stems from reserve with clients. He is not curious about their secrets.

Our challenge is to earn our personhood so that we can live at ease with privacy or openness. When we play an authority role of parenting, supervising, or chairing a committee we must never invade the secrets of others. The Bible's teaching about privacy (e.g., Mark 4:34) commends itself for good sense and workability.

11

Facing Fear

Have no anxiety about anything, but in everything by prayer and supplication with thanksgiving let your requests be made known to God. And the peace of God, which passes all understanding, will keep your hearts and your minds in Christ Jesus (Phil. 4:6-7).

Let me assert my firm belief that the only thing we have to fear is fear itself.

Franklin Delano Roosevelt,
First Inaugural Address
4 March 1933

Perseveration

Today's psychologists say virtually all our emotionally oriented problems relate to a trinity of dragons: guilt, anger, and fear. Guilt is the weight of the past, anger the burden of the present, and fear our worry about the future. Consider these in reverse order.

First we face our anxiety—fear—about the future and seek to find a cure.

113

Perseveration, when used of the brain damaged, refers to uncontrollable rut thinking. Twenty-one-year-old Betty's brain was damaged by a smallpox vaccination in infancy. Betty received a valentine from a secret pal and can't quit talking about it. "Look at my valentine. Who do you think sent it? Doesn't the handwriting look like Auntie Jane's?" On she goes, nonstop, until her parents intervene.

A species of perseveration (pur-sev-er-á-shun) strikes the burnout victim. Insecurity puts a stranglehold on spontaneity, planning suffers paralysis, thought goes in circles.

Fear that one cannot perform at work has become the dynamic. This fear generates preoccupation with details, slows the normal sequence of activity, and interrupts goal achievement.

Almost inevitably this paralysis stems from fear of others. What will the board think? How will the senior partner react? Who will respond negatively? A normal amount of pre-imaging is natural and needed. Carried to extreme, pre-imaging becomes perseveration.

How can we stop? We begin to find the answer in active caring. Face your enemies supposed and real. Do them good professionally and personally. Express your benevolent spirit covertly in words, overtly in cooperative support.

Fear of Failure

On one occasion Steve Allen's interview guest, a doctor, said, "The only two really instinctive fears in men are the fear of loud noises and the fear of falling. What are *you* afraid of?"

"I have a great fear," Allen confessed, "of making a loud noise while falling."

Most of us have conquered the two infancy fears, but anxieties about failure rear their ugly heads in low moments.

We rehearse past mistakes and relive embarrassing events. Usually we can laugh, but in burnout capacities get inhibited. The desk piled with work paralyzes rather than stimulates us to productivity.

How do we get this way? We suffer displeasure with ourselves. The point of unhappiness does not always surface readily and self-preoccupation takes over the search. In this mood we run the risk of inflicting problems and the resultant fears may render us ineffective.

We need not allow these fears and problems to unnerve us. When we find ourselves tempted into the abyss of egocentricity, we can (1) recognize this tendency as a sign. When fatigue threatens us, we do well to attack it. We can help through (2) vigorous exercise like tennis, racquetball, swimming, walking. Caught during the initial stages, fatigue and fear toxins yield to the body's own tranquilizing action. In this relaxed position we can (3) listen to ourselves and expect nature and God to show us the true problem. When the problem is discovered, (4) the mind is content with a moderate appetite for food, drink, and sleep. (Overeating and oversleeping, sometimes undereating and insomnia, are indicators of abnormal emotional involvement.)

Recognition, exercise, listening, and healthy habits go a long way toward coping with the threat of failure.

Overcoming Worry

Worry is a kind of fear. The word comes from the Anglo-Saxon for choke or strangle. This is a clear picture of worry robbing us of full life.

Job 3:25 tells us how worry can work: "For the thing that I fear comes upon me, and what I dread befalls me." Worrywarts get into trouble because trouble gets into them. They attract trouble like a magnet draws filings.

Fear can actually make one choke, like the woman who couldn't swallow. Her pastor worked with her until she saw the psychosomatic dynamics of her worry. Success followed her insight. Choking on food and drink stopped, and normal swallowing returned.

Worry can quickly give us a burned-out feeling, choking life out of us. One cure is to think thoughts antagonistic to worry. Psychologist Aaron Beck handles depression by challenging dark thoughts with their rational opponents. Assert your own views and desires, giving straight-from-the-shoulder "I" messages about your convictions.

We don't have to be rocked back and forth on the sea of worry. We can generate thoughts that create feelings of peace and calm. We can condition ourselves to this style of thinking.

God's promised help in this willful war against worry comes through Isaiah 35:3-4: "Strengthen the weak hands, and make firm the feeble knees. Say to those who are of a fearful heart, 'Be strong, fear not! Behold, your God will come with vengeance, with the recompense of God. He will come and save you.'"

You can take the offensive in these ways: (1) Consciously see yourself conqueror until the subconscious mind makes the spontaneous positive reaction to daily threats. (2) Refuse negative debilitating thoughts. Remember that barely 2 or 3 percent of our anxieties materialize. (3) Remember that God fights for and with us against evil forces. The New Testament says His Spirit lives in us to maintain the victorious abundant life.

Enemies as Opportunities

Enemies unnerve us. We stand in awe, even downright fear, of them. Some enemies are people, some circumstances, others conditions.

116

Our primary challenge relates to attitude. Seeing enemies as opportunities is the secret. Not easy but possible. Thinking demonstrates the power of opposition to prod us into growth and increase our problem-solving skills. Enemies help us see creative possibilities we would otherwise miss, stimulate us to face problems that need solving, and call us to develop strength of character.

This kind of thinking positions us to assume command of problem situations. Fear sets in when 'the enemy' takes command. With clear and sturdy thinking God's Word enables us to live above, not under, our circumstances.

The following methods handle the enemies that can burn and destroy.

See enemies as instruments of your development. See them as friends. E. Stanley Jones believed his critics were the unpaid guardians of his soul. He listened to them, considered carefully their critiques of his ministry, and implemented legitimate suggestions. He grew under criticism. Challenges prevent stunted growth.

See yourself capable of creative coping. God made us bigger than our enemies. His Kingdom within us opens our eyes to varied options, gives a capacity to focus on best choices, and provides energy to implement a determined plan of action. Each of us has far greater potential than we realize available to solve the dilemmas of life.

See your wider opportunities. Intentional prayer, creative listening, innovative design suggest an infinite number of approaches to winning strategies. A telephone call to a wise man put me at ease in a preaching situation where I suspected opposition. I discovered the mind set of the people to whom I had been called to minister.

A carefully planned meeting can yield interest; a well-written letter itemizing precise needs, can bring answers; thoughtfully selected personnel can brainstorm to profit. Part of the fun of living lies in the enormous range of modern technology making new worlds possible to achieve our goals.

Fear of enemies vanishes when we see them as opportunities for growth and achievement.

Attacking Fear with Love

Karl Menninger discovered his clinic produced minimal results. He called his staff together to ask them to add love to their daily rounds. Little deeds of kindness, projections of care and warmth could be evidences of genuine concern. The hospital workers no longer saw patients as mere numbers. Result? Therapy charts showed major improvements in hospital clients.

Dr. Menninger declared, "Love is the medicine for the sickness of the world." His conviction was that the root of most hang-ups centers in the inability to receive or give love. Teach people to love and they live successfully and happily.

Can love handle ordinary everyday fears? Yes. For example, I cannot live in fear of those who genuinely love me, nor will persons fear me for very long if I love them. Even animals respond positively to love, negatively to fear. When I love myself, my fears about myself vanish to bring freedom.

Love replaces fear when we begin with a prayer list of persons for whom we have concern. Love increases for people who have put you off. William Law believed, "There is nothing that makes us love a man so much as praying for him."

Next, pray especially for those who make a point of threatening you. This overt behavior is always a cry for help. Fear responses intensify another's fears. Conversely, love signals put us at ease.

Respond to the imperative call of Ephesians 5:18: ". . . be filled with the Spirit." God's Spirit is love. The first Letter of

One John (4:7-21, e.g.) shows the power of love to overcome fear and maintain Kingdom ideals. Exposure to God, coupled with quiet times facilitate the maintenance of the Spirit of active, expressed love.

Courage

"Screw your courage to a sticking place," cried Lady Macbeth in answer to her husband's fearful question, ". . . if we fail?" Her complete answer exposes her courage. "Screw your courage to the sticking place and we'll not fail."

How do we "screw our courage to the sticking place" in the face of odds bigger than ourselves? When we condition ourselves during calm times we are prepared for rough experiences.

Tenacity develops with finishing tasks. Children need to be taught stick-to-it-iveness. Homework begun must come to completion. Bringing to terminus what we commence builds courage.

Mettle, the ingrained capacity to meet strain and stress, grows by watching examples of courage. Heroic models breed mettle in others. We can model valor, inspiring others.

Resolution to achieve goals comes through practicing a never-say-die behavior. The harder the challenge, the greater girth is added to existing muscle. God calls us to face contests resolutely with His promised help.

Spirit fortifies one to continue against opponents, road blocks, and temptations, and comes from the Spirit of God who is our tenacity, mettle, and resolution. He calls us to depend on Him when we find ourselves up against impossible situations. With reliance comes grace for strengthening.

God's Spirit furnishes courage in the face of fear.

Uses of Fear

Fear has good sides. When threats loom, security comes under seige. Fear has the power to prod us to creative self-defense. Onrushing traffic makes us stop to look both ways.

Fear is ready for translation into good when the latent subconscious impulses threaten to surface and get out of control. For example, anger wells up when a child disobeys or disappoints us because we feel rejected. Our ideals have suffered violation by our own kith and kin. Hurt becomes anger damaging ourselves and our children. Unhappy thoughts need transformation into thoughts of kindness and empathy. God sends His redeeming grace when our wills are set in love.

Fear serves good purposes when it prods us to cry out against evil power structures. When kiddie porn scars innocent minds, we ought to be propelled to act. Interestingly, forthright opposition to evil, flowing from a sure-of-your-ground motivation, does not in itself cause burnout. Withdrawal from confrontation gives rise to guilt and inner conflict, leading to burnout.

Fear your ability to allow love to erode. This happens subtly, as daily life wears thin our genuine affection for others. J. R. Miller, perhaps the most widely read devotional writer of his day, lived for people. As a supervising editor, he even wrote welcome notes to his employees on their return from vacation! As a pastor, he made prospective church members in his catechism class feel important. He was an imaginative Christian worker, with creativity centered in helping individuals. He feared the loss of concern.

In review, fear is constructive when it prompts us to kindness and empathy. It can propel us into battle over specific evils. Constructive fear stimulates us to embrace person-oriented service.

12

Converting Anger

Man who gets angry quickly, gets old quickly.

South Sea Islands proverb

Anger Converted

God designed basic human anger to create good. Rage stimulates the brain, calling for alterations in body chemistry to propel us into remedial action.

A California mother lost her beautiful daughter when a drunk driver used his vehicle as a battering ram. Today that irate mother works effectively with authorities to stop one of the great social evils of our time.

The mother acts wisely, for her redemptive activity serves to bring indignation to resolution. Unresolved anger can build and freeze into depression. It is a major factor in causing burnout.

Unmelted anger can cause illness or contribute to death. A man who bitterly resented his arduous drive to and from daily employment dropped dead on the golf course. No doubt his death came as the result of a complex of reasons, but anger seems to have been one of them.

How can we resolve and convert our anger into something constructive?

Learn to recognize undissolved fury for what it is. Become aware of how anger expresses itself. Freud believed depression was anger turned in on itself, what someone has called frozen rage. Little depressive thoughts and moods may arise from feelings that hide in the subconscious. To become aware of anger's expression is the knowledge that precedes therapeutic action.

Translate your feelings of injustice into constructive activity. People in helping professions object inwardly and angrily to unfairness. They are supposed to, but they dare not leave interior anger boiling. The generated steam needs channeling, like writing an article to clear a misconception, raising tuition money for the young man from deprived circumstances, chairing the local charity committee to correct misallocation of funds.

The Bible admonishes us not to let the sun go down on our wrath. We live fully, says Elisabeth Kübler-Ross, only after getting rid of anger.

Benefits of Hurt and Anger

We know that hurt and anger are close neighbors. Wounds can give birth to anger. Hurt and anger need to be exchanged for peace and love.

How do we exchange the bad feelings for the good?

Recognize the benefits of hurt. "Every wall is a door," said Emerson. Sorrow may be as difficult to break through as the Great Wall of China, but "sorrow is a great revealer." Life is a wall without a door until grief knocks. When we look in the direction of the knock an opening comes into view.

Anger at life's disappointments can blind us to the door in the wall. Conversely, readiness to see reveals the door through which looms a horizon of unspeakable beauty and splendor. Walk through the door into the hope of starting-all-over-again.

Know God stands ready to give you comfort. Jesus announced this truth in a beatitude: "Blessed are they that mourn, for they shall be comforted." Jesus had no doubt about this; God eagerly and readily provides solace when sorrow strikes.

Anger's embrace bars comfort, while a loving soul opens his arms in the presence of Christ to receive consolation.

The Word of God is medicine. Wounds call for treatment. The Bible, known to receptive people for its healing powers, dispenses therapy to hurting people. Written to persons in pain, the Scriptures breathe the very healing power of God.

When hurt and angry, experiment in a quiet place with meditation. Read the open Book. Watch clouds lift. Observe your return to normalcy. Ponder the fresh insights that come from the Medicine of Truth.

Healers Get Healed

Modern psychiatry tells us deeply hurt persons work through anger very slowly. Acts of love can assist and hasten the process. A loving lifestyle gives a daily therapy to hurting people, averting anger build-up.

The selfless turning away from our own injustices to concentration on others has great power to heal. *Healers get healed.*

A pastor who studies the art of kindness fills his days ministering to bring relief. He does favors for the unloved and lonely, a short note to one in grief, a call requiring counsel to put into motion comforting and strengthening influences. No wonder he sleeps soundly at night.

The genius of kindness is self-giving. A mental patient rejected her young chaplain's offer of candy because she sensed the chocolates served as a substitute for giving himself. Jesus gave no money, food, or clothes. He detected deeper hungers for love and longing for companionship. Jesus met these elemental needs for friendship not by activism, but by the simple ministry of presence. He showed interest in people which made them feel worthwhile. Gentleness, a caring spirit, concern, and empathy all speak eloquently from our Lord's life.

A recent theorist about teenage suicide states that anger at God gets at the root cause of self-destruction. "Why have you made me this way? Why have you put me in this environment? Why have you created me at all?" Suicide is the ultimate revenge against the Creator.

We can bring moderating influences to bear on despondent lives, sometimes making a heaven out of a hell. This service won't make a headline, but it can translate someone's restlessness into calm and blackness into sunshine. In the process our own anger, self-pity, and egocentricity is released.

Anger and a New Job

The average American changes jobs ten times in the course of his life. Anger sometimes raises its ugly head when one changes position.

Change breeds insecurity; job stability fosters (too easily) security. Adjustments drain energies, and if input does not keep pace with emotional investment, burnout may ensue.

Sometimes an administrator or overseer sees you more advantageously placed in another role. The alteration may cause you a bit of torment and paranoia. Work through the anger as quickly as possible, and get on with the new responsibilities. St. John of the cross advised us to pay as little attention as possible to hurts.

Occasionally a fresh opportunity requires moving to another place. The mobility rate charts in the United States reflect high turnovers; some communities have very high percentages. Children suffer as they leave friends and a happy school behind. Wives chafe under the necessity of settling into a different home. Family finances suffer in the buying and selling of real estate. Adjustments to the local cost-of-living index can prove more challenging than one would like. A new atmosphere calls for coping with requirements of the different environment.

Short-fused people find adjustment hard. Christian disciplines and God's grace provide the grand sources of help.

The exercise of faith means tapping expedient resources. You *remember* (an important word in the Bible) God's effective help in the past, and know He will not forget you now. In this move, with its variables, you realize His grand blueprint for your life moves a step further down the road to fulfillment. God is your Father, who dependably guides and provides for you.

Mind-stretching stimulations to faith are based solidly on God's Word and Christian experience. They bring growth, invigorating strength, and the comfort characterized in the word *paraclete*, the One alongside us.

Tackling Leader Isolation

Leaders suffer isolation for many reasons. They may think ahead of others, therefore separating themselves to some degree. They dream great dreams, making some preoccupied with daily duties feel inferior. Leaders who serve well listen carefully, but others may feel so threatened they cannot listen easily. Leaders accept people and try to empathize. Few followers fully accept and identify with authority figures.

Leaders suffer isolation. Rage may accumulate when they are pushed out of the normal social circle. Leaders must pretend they're okay all the time. Some professionals busy themselves to drown the sense of exile. Others turn to drink or drugs, with worse imprisonment. Others seek contact by a kind of desperate talkativeness, only to find ostracism increased.

All negative techniques end in double failure: isolation worsens, anger accumulates. How do we cope with isolation?

Accept it as the price of leadership. No position in life frees one entirely of problems. Those who cannot tolerate the difficulties of leadership do not thrill to the excitements of high challenge. Moreover, expertise requires a certain solitude; the resultant elevation and authority mean separated existence.

Remind yourself that rewards do come. The listening, loving, sympathetic leader receives great honor and respect. The loyalty followers express in gifts, banquet speeches, appreciation notes, a knowing handshake is touching. Depend on this law of life, loving leaders get love in return. Love may come back only after years of personal investment, sometimes through the most trying of circumstances, but some day affection will ride in on a handsome horse. That reality does a lot to deflate the sense of loneliness.

Push others up the ladder. Wise preachers invite the best guest preachers, seek advice from persons of knowledge, hand responsibility over to potential leaders. The confidence born in persons who feel important generates warm friendships. The rich fellowship that follows helps meet one's own felt needs.

The Focus Was Christ

In February, 1982, I listened to a black man from Uganda tell the story of the East Africa Revival. The talk took place at the Evangelical Bible Seminary of Southern Africa, Pietermaritzburg, South Africa. I saw the power of God to handle anger in special circumstances.

The story began in the late 1920s and early '30s when spiritual problems mounted so high that missionaries wanted to go home. Gospel workers felt depressed, angry, and burned out.

In 1935 a black man and a white man, studying Scripture together, experienced a genuine revelation. Through the cross and confession of their sins, they could be victorious over sin.

This illuminating discovery took revival dimensions. Whole nights of prayer, a spirit of oneness in Christ, multiplied conversions among Australians, Germans, and others then in East Africa, was accompanied by a remarkable variety of other miracles.

The hallmark of the revival, which continues to this day, is Jesus. He is central—not miracles of healing, or gifts of the Spirit, or any other manifestation. Jesus is everything.

In Him lies the secret. Focus on gifts, and jealousies well up. Zero in on healing, and arguments emerge. Put persons in the limelight, and hearts give birth to antagonisms. When the focus is on anything but Christ the sprouting of anger produces a crop of hate.

Christ is freedom from anger. We make Him central by (1) willfully putting and keeping Him there. This is an act of the will. This is also a (2) daily decision. Expose yourself to influences that facilitate regular decisiveness: Bible meditation, devotional enlightenment, Christian conversation.

The centralizing of Christ becomes the pivot of a lifestyle. (3) The Christ-centered style yields growth which means stamina. There is openness to the continuing and deepening purification of His Spirit through this Jesus centrality.

The East Africa Revival

The Jesus revival in East Africa had definite characteristics.

Walking in the light. Christians kept a clean conscience before God and one another. Pride, jealousy with sins of thought and behavior came to confession. Hiding from one's offenses simply was not done. When one walked in darkness unwittingly, the Spirit turned light on the sin. Revealed, the moral violation came under intense internal censure, confession followed, then forgiveness.

Restitution. Converted Christians returned stolen items. Shocked authorities listened to accounts of misbehavior. Grateful businessmen collected overdue monies. In every case of restitution, miracles of transformation and good will were taking place.

Brokenness. To receive criticism graciously is genuine humility. Preachers took corrections, Gospel workers submitted to admonitions, husbands and wives surrendered their differences and found reconciliation. In such a Spirit-oriented environment, hostilities simply did not have a chance to build up.

The cross of Christ. The Gospel accounts of Jesus' finished work communicated with astonishing impact to all Spirit-filled Christians. The availability of atonement for cleansing the human heart and sustaining that cleansing, made its New Testament impression on sincere persons.

When this biblical Christianity invades a soul distraught by injustices and depressions, renewal sets in. Anyone experienced in vital Christianity knows the reality of erased resentments and the resulting sense of relief.

The radical and divine remedy for anger is awareness of sin, restitution, and holy forgiveness.

13

Dealing with Guilt

A man can stand a lot as long as he can stand himself. He can live without hope, without books, without friends, without music as long as he can listen to his own thoughts.

Axel Munthe
The Story of San Michele

Perspective

We come now to the third dragon, guilt. The first, fear, is the burden of the future; the second, anger, is the weight of the present; the third, guilt, is the concern we carry about the past.

Initially, we need to remind ourselves of the difference between guilt and guilt feelings. Real guilt centers in wrongs actually done, objective sin. Guilt feelings may or may not find their source in moral wrongdoing. Everyone does not have a conscience about violating God's laws. Some sense guilt when they have done nothing amiss. Conscientious persons can wrongly carry a load of guilt if they cannot go to every meeting, see everyone who calls, and contribute to every worthy cause.

Elisabeth Kübler-Ross dedicates her life to relieving the fear and guilt of those who are dying. She believes natively happy children in the West get contaminated as they grow, developing false guilts. The purpose of medicine, in her view, is to release persons from damaging guilt feelings.

Get real guilt sorted out from mere, unnecessary guilty feelings. Find a New Testament perspective through honesty, evaluation, and God's grace.

Honesty. List your supposed wrongdoings. Eliminate what you only imagine as integrity breaks, testing uncertainties against Scripture. Bring obvious sins to God. Take as long as you need to assess your moral status but clear your conscience. The resulting peace makes the effort vastly worthwhile.

Evaluation. Arriving at a realistic perspective revolves around complex factors. A young college professor, in charge of a small account, spent money from the fund on a project, then had second thoughts. Did he misappropriate funds? Wisely he spoke to his superior to clear the matter and his conscience returned to rest. Get the kind of help you need with ethically gray questions. Responsible evaluation allows the mind to rest.

God's grace. Some wrongdoing cannot undergo evaluation because time and distance preclude clearing the air. Only the rain of grace can create a fresh atmosphere for the soul to live and breathe freely. Sincere, guileless Christians find God's grace operative for particular and specific needs.

Whatever the cost, establish perspective.

Freedom

The Axel Munthe quotation on the title page of this section on guilt inadvertently reveals the grand freedom of one who lives the forgiven life. Feel yourself recover from fatigue when you enjoy the liberty of a clear, clean conscience.

Munthe's four illustrations may be therapeutic instruments with peculiar power to work for minds free of guilt.

Hope. Hopeful minds exude optimism while guilty minds emit pessimism. There was a Christian who had cheated on his wife. He tried to cover his sin, arguing the obsolescence of the "old" morality. Nothing in his life worked happily, not his job, his social relationships, or his plans. All took on dull coloration. Neither counseling nor medication put vibrancy back into life. When he faced sin, confessed it, received divine forgiveness, and started all over again, he began to live comfortably with himself.

Books. Try to absorb yourself in a book when guilt courses down the runways of your mind. Perhaps for a little while one can escape in reading, but the culpability threat always returns. The mind free to enter into a writer's creativity finds diversion and has liberty to restore itself.

Friends. "You can't find anything better for beating fatigue," said an observer at a house party. Fun, food, fellowship have almost magical restorative powers. This medication does its fullest work for free persons. The person fighting guilt remains unrestored.

Music. Nothing captures one's soul like a Mozart symphony or a Vivaldi chamber work. Folk tunes have power to express our feelings about the past, conjuring nostalgia. Music is such a powerful healing tool that a whole new therapeutic movement centers around it.

Forgiven persons enjoy freedom to use God's instruments of hope, books, friends, and music to achieve wholeness.

Subconscious Guilt

A major factor in burnout is guilt hidden in the subconscious mind. Vague hints surface now and again while undefined floating anxieties pester us. Some of these unconscious guilts come from cultural sins, like manipulation.

Manipulating people, robbing them of information, and slanting data, renders us dishonest. In quiet moments we envision the ultimate implications and fear them. Because culture accepts and hides manipulation, we talk ourselves out of facing the issues.

We do not verbalize these thoughts but we have them. They irritate because the radicality of the Gospel gets through every time we read the New Testament. We need to halt our guilt.

Invite the Spirit of God to make us vividly aware of New Testament ethics. Little by little the Spirit shows motivations that characterize interpersonal relations. He gets more specific about the way we spend money. One of the best guides to uncovering personal biblical ethics is Richard J. Foster's *Freedom of Simplicity.* Dr. Foster faces the difficulties while refusing to give an inch on the real issues. We become alive to the truth that hurts us.

Implement your emerging awarenesses. Suppose I discover racial prejudice in myself. I had thought I enjoyed freedom from that sin; now I discover superiority feelings toward other peoples. I see my American way as being above, for example, African ways. I begin to read, gather information, and analyze myself critically. Finally the Spirit tells me specific ways I can put into action my dawning revelations.

Detecting hidden guilt and accepting it can be a major step to recovery and renewal. O. Hobart Mowrer observed that one who lives "under the shadow of real, unacknowledged and unexpiated guilt . . . will continue to hate himself and to suffer the inevitable consequences of self-hatred."

Mowrer goes on to declare that the moment one "begins to accept his guilt and his sinfulness, the possibility of radical reformation opens up, and a new freedom of self-respect and peace."

The Untidy Conscience

John Woolman, eighteenth-century American Quaker, had forthright courageous convictions that made a difference. His belief in simplicity continues to challenge and influence the shape of our stewardship. His rugged personal honesty set in motion ripples that continue. His quiet fight against slavery brought a halt to that despicable sin among Friends long before the Civil War. By 1770 no Quaker kept slaves.

Woolman had little going for him. He lived only fifty-two years, never possessed the skill to organize a typical American protest movement. He didn't even have the physical strength to match his challenges. Yet he achieved substantial goals.

He refused to live with an untidy conscience. To see a fellow human being in need was an occasion to meet that need whatever the inconvenience. In his *Plea for the Poor*, he recommends work with the poverty stricken to identify with their plight.

He shaped his lifestyle to his calling. This Quaker tailor cut off opportunities to develop his business for a number of reasons, one of the most important being to make possible the traveling ministry to which God called him. He lived on a meager income and determined nothing would hinder completion of his divine assignments. He deliberately refused fame and fortune to follow the Inner Light. He refers to being "weaned from the desire of outward greatness" and silencing "every motion proceeding from the love of money."

He spoke strongly against evil. His protests were not always verbal. He might quietly walk away from his noon meal to protest to a family keeping a slave. He refused to make out a receipt for the sale of a black man. When he did speak in uncensuring tones, he offered probing questions to slave owners. What happens to you as a moral person when you keep slaves? What kind of moral education do you model for your children? For thirty years John Woolman rode his horse up and down the East coast, pressing moral claims in his own calm and persistent way.

Woolman listened to the Inner Voice. He developed a conscience sensitive to human need. He discovered a profoundly effective preventative medicine against guilt.

"Cumbers"

John Woolman called incumbrances "cumbers." These burdens of guilt need to be unloaded so the heaviness does not create a type of burnout. God calls us to give Him our cumbers: ". . . let us also lay aside every weight . . ." (Heb. 12:1).

Look at two cumbers.

Using instead of building people. Robert K. Greenleaf, in *Servant Leadership*, observes that some leaders see institutions as people developers. Persons "grow taller and become healthier, stronger, more autonomous." Other leaders use persons as devices to make the institution grow. Greenleaf rightly observes that the latter leaders succeed only for a time while the others endure.

Get rid of the people-using cumber and find a new measure of release from guilt.

Doing what looks good instead of what is good. Each person has different needs and serves God in his or her own way. Only God and oneself can judge what lies behind appearances. The biblically oriented person knows when he spends time, money, and talent in the true interests of God and man.

Elton Trueblood describes on-the-spot research about conversion. When twenty-five persons were asked how they met Christ, they indicated that an ordinary person served as the instrument. None of the twenty-five referred to a big public presentation or conspicuous soul-winning. God uses the humble to get His work done.

Content yourself with inconspicuous servanthood and watch the burden of "significance," fraught with guilt overtones, fall away.

These items suggest the kind of temptations we struggle against. Willingness to confront temptation leads to unloading the guilt. Temple Gairdner counseled about getting rid of one kind of temptation this way: "take it out into the desert with Christ and throttle it!"

A Jewish legend says when Satan was asked what he missed most about heaven, he replied, "the trumpets in the morning." Burnout victims suffer low enthusiasm. Ridding ourselves of cumbers opens our soul's eyes to a fresh vision of inspiration. When we hear trumpets in the morning we know that God has done something with our guilt.

Healing for Guilt

Whether guilt feelings issue from concern about objective wrongdoing, imagined guilt, or a sense of guilt about feeling guilty, God provides healing and release. Here are three divine antidotes.

The healing sacraments. The Christian saints through the centuries commend, sometimes in strong language, the sacraments for those in need of spiritual freedom. They see the danger of pride, source of all sin, and therefore root of guilt and guilt feelings. They recognize isolationist tendencies in those who center on God in dead earnest. They know the necessity of the solitary life which fosters unreal perceptions. Whenever one takes the Lord's Supper or participates in a service of baptism (or re-lives his or her baptism), the Body of Christ comes alive. Christ Himself is present to bring healing through the restoration of perspective and the forgiveness of sins. He presents Himself for healing.

The healing Word. Martin Luther insisted that the spoken Word frees and sustains us. By listening to the preached Word the Church finds nourishment and preservation. Luther said our souls can do without anything except God's Word, which provides truth, light, peace, righteousness, salvation, joy, and liberty. When we hear and believe the Word centered in Christ, we are fed, made righteous, set free, and made whole. Healthy Christians are healthy precisely because their guilts are exposed to God's Word spoken by the power of the Spirit who releases us.

A healing friend. A Celtic proverb hits the nail on the head:

> Anyone without a soul friend
> is a body without a head.

Aelred of Rievaulx agreed that friendship was essential. Living without friends is living like a beast. Friendship is a steppingstone to bring us up to the love and knowledge of God . . . "friendship lies close to perfection." Our greatest mistake is to believe we can be free of guilt and guilt feelings without confiding in a trusted friend, pastor, spouse, or prayer partner. Talking in a conducive atmosphere opens the door to the Spirit's clarifying, forgiving, and therapeutic ministries.

Elisabeth Kübler-Ross expresses surprise at the number of honorary doctorates universities have given her. "I don't understand this, all I've done is listen to people." Quite enough, Dr. Kübler-Ross, quite enough.

The Impact of Guilt and Release

Freud taught the need to get rid of guilt, which he said served as a deterrent to health. Pathological guilt does, but the recognition of sin with accompanying guilt feelings is enormously healthy, a sign of the work of the Holy Spirit.

Carl Menninger defined sin as "at heart a refusal of the love of others." Every time we get a fresh glimpse of how to love others better, we experience both sadness and elation. Sadness or guilt because we see our neglect; elation because we discover new ways to improve relationships.

An essential problem with some therapeutic theories is a disease mentality. Any therapy foundation that works from a disease as over against a health model, results in twisted thinking. Concentration on guilt will not make it disappear. Submerging guilt leaves it to fester and erupt in ugly expressions. Who can deny the social and emotional impact of guilt?

Some try to deny guilt by doing sins that create bad feelings. This kind of whistling in the dark does not expel the bogeyman. Others point to social influences that condition conscience. They ignore the moral "ought" created in people. All denial is theological. We cannot live against the God inside us without suffering serious consequences.

To live in cooperation with the God inside results in enormous energy. That energy, moral- and value-oriented, means creativity instead of staleness, flexibility instead of rigidity, possibilities instead of paralysis, love instead of fear, integration instead of splintering, worship instead of self-preoccupation, joy instead of injury, laughter instead of depression.

Bibliography

à Kempis, Thomas, *Imitation of Christ* put into contemporary English format by Donald E. Demaray. Grand Rapids: Baker Book House, 1982.

Aquinas, Thomas, *My Way of Life: The Summa Simplified for Everyone* by Walter Farrell and Martin J. Healy. Brooklyn: Confraternity of the Precious Blood, 1952.

Allen, David E., and Lewis P. Bird and Robert Herrmann, Editors, *Whole-Person Medicine: An International Symposium*. Downers Grove, Ill.: Inter-Varsity Press, 1980.

"America Shapes Up," *Time*, November 2, 1981.

Badham, Leslie, *Verdict on Jesus*. London: Hodder and Stoughton, 1971.

Barzun, Jacques, Editor, *Pleasures of Music: An Anthology about Music and Musicians*. London: Cassell, 1977 edition; Chicago: University of Chicago Press, 1977.

Benson, Dale, *The Total Man*. Wheaton: Tyndale, 1977.

Bombeck, Erma, *Aunt Erma's Cope Book*. New York: Fawcett, 1981 (pb).

Brinsmead, Robert D., *This Is Life*. Fallbrook, California: Verdict Publications, 1978.

Cousins, Norman, *Anatomy of an Illness as Perceived by the Patient*. New York: W. W. Norton and Co., 1979.

————, *Human Options*. New York: Norton, 1981.

Drucker, Peter F., "Know Thy Time," *Leadership*, Spring 1982.

Engstrom, Ted W., and Edward R. Dayton, *Christian Leadership Newsletter*. Monrovia: World Vision.

Engstrom, Ted W., and Edward R. Dayton, "Time for Things that Matter," *Leadership*, Spring 1982.

Engstrom, Ted W., and David J. Juroe, *The Work Trap*. Old Tappan, N.J.: Fleming H. Revell, 1979.

Foster, Richard J., *Celebration of Discipline: The Path to Spiritual Growth.* New York: Harper and Row, 1978.

―――――, *Freedom of Simplicity.* New York: Harper and Row, 1981.

Freudenberger, Herbert J., and Geraldine Richelson, *Burn-Out: The High Cost of High Achievement.* Garden City, New York: Doubleday, 1981.

Fullam, Everett L., *Living the Lord's Prayer.* Lincoln, Va.: Chosen Books, 1980.

Gardner, John W., *Self-Renewal: The Individual and the Innovative Society.* New York: Harper and Row, 1963.

Greenleaf, Robert K., *Servant Leadership.* New York: Paulist Press, 1977.

Hammarskjöld, Dag, *Markings,* translated by Leif Sjöberg and W. H. Auden. London: Faber and Faber, 1966 (9th edition pb).

"Headache Sufferers: Help Is on the Way," An interview with Dr. David R. Coddon, *U.S. News and World Report,* May 24, 1982.

"Job Burnout: Growing Worry for Workers, Bosses," An interview with Cary Cherniss. *U.S. News and World Report,* February 18, 1980.

Jones, E. Stanley, *Abundant Living.* Nashville: Abingdon Festival Books, 1976 (pb).

―――――, *Christian Maturity.* Nashville: Abingdon Festival Books, 1980 (pb).

―――――, *Growing Spiritually.* Nashville: Abingdon Festival Books, 1978 (pb).

Kehl, D. G., "Burnout: The Risk of Reaching Too High," *Christianity Today,* November 20, 1981.

Kennedy, Marilyn Moats, *Career Knockouts: How to Battle Back.* New York: Warner Books, 1979.

Larson, Bruce, *There's a Lot More to Health Than Not Being Sick.* Waco: Word Books, 1981.

Laubach, Frank C., *Letters by a Modern Mystic.* Westwood, N.J.: Fleming H. Revell, 1958.

Leech, Kenneth, *Soul Friend: A Study in Spirituality.* London: Sheldon Press, 1977; New York: Harper and Row, 1980.

―――――, *True Prayer, an Invitation to Christian Spirituality.* New York: Harper and Row, 1981.

Maddocks, Morris, *The Christian Healing Ministry.* London: SPCK, 1981.

Mesmer, Robert, M.D., "Burnout: Its Relevance to the Christian Physician," *Christian Medical Society Journal.* January 1982.

Morley, Robert, *Book of Worries.* London: Weidenfeld and Nicolson, 1979; Hollywood: Warner Books, 1981 (pb).

"Nutritional Psychosis," *Omni,* vol. 4, no. 8.

Peale, Norman Vincent, *Dynamic Imaging: The Powerful Way to Change Your Life.* Old Tappan, N.J.: Fleming H. Revell, 1982.

―――――, *Stay Alive All Your Life.* New York: Fawcett, 1978 (pb).

Potter, Beverly, *Beating Job Burnout.* New York: Ace Books, 1980.

Rooney, Andy, *A Few Minutes with Andy Rooney.* New York: Atheneum, 1981.

"Salt: A New Villain?" *Time,* March 15, 1982.

Selye, Hans, M.D., *The Stress of Life.* New York: McGraw Hill, 1976 (revised).

————, *Stress Without Distress.* Philadelphia: J.B. Lippincott, 1974.

Shedd, Charlie W., *Time for All Things: Meditations on the Christian Management of Time.* Nashville: Abingdon Press, Apex edition, 1972.

Stein, Kathleen, "Dr. C's Vitamin Elixers," *Omni,* vol. 4, no. 7.

Taylor, Cedric, and Graeme Goldsworthy, *Battle Guide for Christian Leaders, An Endangered Species.* Cudgen, N.S.W. 2413, Australia: Wellcare Publications, 1981.

Teresa, Mother of Calcutta, *A Gift for God.* New York: Harper and Row, 1975.

Tournier, Paul, *Secrets* (tr. by Joe Embry). Richmond, Va.: John Knox Press, 1965.

Trobisch, Walter, *I Married You.* New York: Harper and Row, 1975 (pb).

Veninga, Robert, and James Spradley, "How to Cope with Job Burnout," *Reader's Digest,* February 1982.